THE EMBODIMENT OF MIND: EASTERN AND WESTERN PERSPECTIVES

THE EMBODIMENT OF MIND: EASTERN AND WESTERN PERSPECTIVES

M.M. DelMonte, Ph.D. & Y. Haruki, Ph.D.
(Editors)

Eburon Publishers, Delft

Also available in this series of publications:

- Y. Haruki, Y. Ishii & M. Suzuki (eds.)
  Comparative and Psychological Study on Meditation (ISBN 90-5166-483-4).
- M.G.T. Kwee & T.L. Holdstock (eds.)
  Western and Buddhist Psychology. Clinical Perspectives (ISBN 90-5166-477-X).

Order from your local bookstore or directly from Eburon:
by fax (31-15-2146888) or
E-mail (info@eburon.nl)

ISBN 90-5166-638-1

Published in the Netherlands by
Eburon Publishers
P.O. Box 2867
NL-2601 CW Delft
E-mail: info@eburon.nl

TABLE OF CONTENTS

PREFACE

This book contains the proceedings of two professional meetings organised by "The Transnational Network for the Study of Physical, Psychological and Spiritual Well-being". Professor Yutaka Haruki is overall convenor of this Network. Both meetings took place in or near Montreal, Canada, in August 1996.

Part I of this book is edited by Dr. Michael M. DelMonte. It contains papers presented at a conference chaired and convened by Dr. DelMonte and entitled "Body over Mind or Mind over Body: Does it Matter? This conference was held at the Manoir d'Youville, Chateauquay, Quebec from 12th to 15th August 1996. It was conjointly organised by Dr. Michael DelMonte, Professor Yutaka Haruki and Mr. Mark Blows.

We are very grateful to the Grey Nuns of Manoir d'Youville and in particular to Sister Doreen Romandini for providing such an idyllic island setting for the conference.

Part II of this book is conjointly edited by Professor Yutaka Haruki and Dr. Michael DelMonte. It contains papers presented at a symposium convened and chaired by Professor Yutaka Haruki and Dr. Jon Kabat Zinn entitled "Does the Concept of Embodiment offer Something New in Psychology?" The symposium took place on 20th August 1996 at the XXVI International Congress of Psychology in Montreal.

Neither of these two meetings would have been possible without the very generous financial assistance organised by Professor Haruki. We wish to express our deep gratitude for this funding, which was provided by the Ibuka Fund of Waseda University, Tokyo. We also would like to offer special thanks to Mark Blows, who, as is his wont with our Network projects, ensured with his abundant enthusiastic support, that we would make a success of this conjoint venture. Last, but not least a final word of thanks to Dr. Maurits Kwee for his helpful advice and support in publishing this material.

Michael M. DelMonte
St. Patrick's Hospital
Dublin, Ireland

and

Yutaka Haruki
Waseda University
Tokyo, Japan

LIST OF CONTRIBUTORS

1. Mark W. Blows, M.A.(Hons.)
   Clinical Psychologist
   Private Practice
   Kenthurst, N.S.W.
   Australia

2. Michael M. DelMonte, Ph.D.
   Senior Clinical Psychologist
   St. Patrick's Hospital
   Dublin 8
   Ireland

3. Padmal de Silva, F.B.Ps.S., C.Psychol.
   Senior Lecturer & Consultant
   Clinical Psychologist
   The Maudsley
   Institute of Psychiatry
   University of London
   England

4. Yutaka Haruki, Ph.D.
   Professor of Psychology
   School of Human Sciences
   Waseda University
   Tokorozawa
   Japan

5. Yoshitaka Konno, Ph.D.
   Professor of Psychology
   Faculty of Human Science
   Bunkyo University
   Japan

6. Maurits G.T. Kwee, Ph.D.
   Head of Behavioural Psychotherapy
   Senior Clinical Psychologist
   Joris Psychiatric Centre
   Delft
   The Netherlands

7. Kiyotaka Mayazaki, M.A.
Associate Professor of Psychology
School of Human Sciences
Waseda University
Tokorozawa
Japan

8. Candace B. Pert, Ph.D.
Research Professor
Department of Physiology & Biophysics
School of Medicine
Georgetown University
Washington D.C.
U.S.A.

9. Yosuke Sakairi, M.A.
Associate Professor of Clinical Psychology
Tokoha Gakuen University
Shizuoka
Japan

10. Saroja Srinivasan, Ph.D.
Clinical Psychologist
Psycnet, Psychology Consultants
Sydney
Australia

11. Elisabeth A. Stutchbury, Ph.D.
Department of Anthropology
Australian National University
Canberra
Australia

12. S. Kay Toombs, Ph.D.
Associate Professor of Philosophy
Philosophy Department
Baylor University
Waco, Texas
U.S.A.

13. Nicole Tremblay, Ph.D.
Clinical Psychologist
Private Practice
Quebec
Canada

14. Weidong Wang, M.A.,
Associate Professor of Chinese Medicine
Guang An Men Hospital
China Academy of Traditional
Chinese Medicine
Beijing
China

FOREWORD

As is obvious from the list of contributors, they come from a variety of professional backgrounds, but most are either academic or clinical psychologists. However, there are also noteworthy contributions from a physiologist, an anthropologist, a philosopher and a practitioner of traditional Chinese medicine. All of the contributors share a strong interest in the mind-brain debate, but naturally approach the issue from different perspectives.

The papers appear in the order in which they were presented. It was decided not to group them into theoretical, clinical and research sub-sections as the great majority of the papers are theoretical and/or descriptive. There are two research papers (i.e. by Dr. Sakairi and Dr. Konno). A few papers contain varying amounts of clinical material alongside their theoretical content (e.g. in the presentations of Dr. Kwee, Dr. Srinivasan and Dr. DelMonte). It is hoped that this collection will stimulate further theorising and research into the mind-body debate, and that such a debate will not only be inter-disciplinary but will also include both Eastern and Western perspectives.

Western psychology has been dominated by the "logical positivism" propounded by Auguste Compte, and tends to confine its range of application to that which is observable, measurable and repeatable. This empirical approach has its undoubted value but so has the much more ancient approach based on the Wisdom Traditions of the Orient. For example, Western psychologists typically tend to operate "from the head" and, as with cognitive therapy, use reason and logic to solve emotional problems.

The Eastern traditions, as in Zen, Yoga and Aikido for example, place considerable value on working from the body, and are less likely to use a rational "talking cure" approach. In fact, in meditation the role of language is entirely side-stepped and silence is seen as playing a central role in emotional healing and growth. These and other related issues will be elaborated in the very stimulating papers which follow.

Michael DelMonte
St. Patrick's Hospital
Dublin 8
Ireland

PART I

CONFERENCE ORGANISED BY THE TRANSNATIONAL NETWORK FOR THE STUDY OF PHYSICAL, PSYCHOLOGICAL AND SPIRITUAL WELL-BEING, ENTITLED: "BODY OVER MIND: DOES IT MATTER?"

Michael M. DelMonte
Convenor, Chairman and Editor

12th - 15th August, 1996

Manoir d'Youville
Chateauquay
Quebec
Canada

WHAT KIND OF DISCIPLINE IS THE BODY/MIND PROBLEM ?

Opening Adress to the 3rd Conference of the Transnational Network for the Study of Physical, Psychological and Spiritual Wellbeing-at Manoir D'Youville, Chateauguay, Quebec, Yutaka Haruki, Ph. D., Professor of Psychology, Waseda University, Japan

The modern science known today as "Psychology" began and subsequently developed in the Occident. No such psychology really took root in the Orient, however. The current psychology practiced in today's Orient is a transplant from the West, and there isn't any psychology that could be called endemic to the East.

However, it goes without saying that the peoples of the East have extensively contemplated the mind and body of the human being. There are several reasons why this did not take shape in anything resembling traditional Western psychology. The largest reason is that Eastern people did not adopt a thought process characterized by analysis and reductionism which has prevailed in the West. This is attributed to the fact that they adopted a holistic frame, which is to say, they always considered the entire phenomenon. Therefore, when they pondered the human mind, the body was also included in their thinking, and likewise, when the body was the object of consideration, the relationship to the mind was also brought to bear.

In the West, when one thinks about the mind and body, greater value is placed on the mind, supposing that the body should be controlled by, or subjected to the mind. In stark contrast to this, the East gave no thought to the dominance or inferiority of either the mind or the body. Rather than trying to find a solution to problems of the mind, they looked to the body, and for solutions to problems with the human body, they turned to the mind. This is due to the emphasis they placed on the value of the body in relationship to the mind, rather than isolating the mind, and considering it an entity unto itself.

Therefore, if psychology can be assumed to be nothing more than a scientific method that only concerns itself with the human mind, then the Eastern approach, at least in so far as the sort of approach centered around China is concerned, can not really be called psychology. (India might be close to the West on this point, however). If we assume that psychology is a discipline that develops techniques that solve problems of the human mind and body, then a merging of the East and West is conceivable. However, such a discipline would no longer be labelled as "psychology". Neither would it fall under existing notions of religion or philosophy. It will undoubtedly be the impending combination of Eastern and Western learning that answers the question, "Then just what kind of discipline is it ?"

It is my hope that this conference will help give rise to a new paradigm on how to regard the mind and the body.

THE MIND VERSUS MATTER DEBATE

Michael M. DelMonte, M.Sc., M. Sc. Psych., Ph.D.,
Senior Clinical Psychologist, St. Patrick's Hospital, Dublin, Ireland

I would like to start at the beginning, i.e. with the emergence of life on earth. When we talk about the origin of life we normally have in mind its biological beginnings and manifestations. The public position held by many, if not most, scientists (e.g. Reville, 1996) is that life emerged as the result of chemical evolution. There is little or no disagreement that some simple chemicals like hydrogen "evolved" into more complex elements via nuclear fusion. However, it is further argued that certain essential carbon compounds arose "by chance", and gradually developed or evolved into more complex chemicals capable of self-replication.

The apparent public consensus in the scientific community as to the origin of life may be considerably weaker when scientists discuss these matters in private. Precisely how ordinary matter became animated by the "vital energy" that distinguishes living matter from inanimate chemical matter is unknown. Likewise, the question as to why this vital animation should have occurred at all leaves practically all scientists puzzled. Bringing God into the equation hardly smacks of "hard science", and tends to embarrass most of us even more than the opportunistic use of the convenient metaphor "by chance".

It is in the main agreed that the biological manifestations of life could have evolved only under certain fairly narrowly defined conditions. In other words, many complex laws of physics operated within *very narrow parameters* in order to produce and sustain living matter. Even *small* deviations in any one of these would have spelled disaster in the tentative and delicate evolution of life. However, the view that all of these prerequisites came together simply "by chance" is disputable and rather meaningless conjecture, with broader implications to which I shall return later.

The principles of contemporary neuro-biology are ultimately based on the theory of genetic evolution. Evolutionary complexification operates *against* entropy, i.e. against the general tendency towards *disorder* (the Second Law of Thermo-dynamics). Yet, despite this, mind is seen by some scientists as only a secondary epiphenomenon, spontaneously emergent out of biological matter in general and out of our operative brains in particular. In other words, for many neuro-biologists mind is the innocent by-product of the brain in action - which in turn was produced fortuitously, i.e. unprompted, *against* the forces of entropy! So with this view, life arose casually as a purely chemical and biological phenomenon; and subsequently mind somehow came to inhabit complex biological matter in just as mysterious a manner as life previously came to animate inorganic matter!

We can thus summarise the "received wisdom" on the origins of life as follows: Inorganic matter somehow evolved into simple *living* matter (vitilisation), and living matter somehow evolved into more complex *conscious* matter (mentalisation), culminating in humans capable of self-reflection (and spirituality?). But how and why?

Some authors, e.g. Pierre Teilhard de Chardin (1965) and, in his own way, Carl Jung (1958), have envisaged the above relationship the other way around; namely, unmanifest "universal mind" exists independently of matter, and it shapes evolution insofar as the evolutionary process and the resultant biological diversity and sophistication reflect universal mind. In other words, from the above perspective universal mind "uses" the physical (and organic) domain to express itself - right down to the level of embodied "personal mind". The latter, with its individual consciousness, is also referred to as the psyche. This is another way of saying that matter is "bathed" in (universal) mind - rather than mind being solely confined to living matter. Variations in nervous systems would affect the organisms' ability to "tune into" universal mind.

However, when we look at life through the confined lenses of neuro-biology then diverse phenomena such as music, painting, dance, poetry, literature, mathematics, architecture, etc., are just envisaged as by-products of the complex workings of human brains which, as already mentioned, purportedly developed "by chance". Put differently, human life and all its cultural manifestations are an "accident" of bio-chemical evolution and have *no meaning* per se. With this model there is an implied primacy of matter over mind, i.e. mind is matter-made - with "man-made" mind being its ultimate expression!

Theories of biological evolution are based on the environmental selection of the fittest genes. Such selection is not seen to be guided by any purpose - spiritual or otherwise. This biological focus betrays a split between material manifestations of life and those domains (e.g. psychic and spiritual) which lie beyond the level of appearances. When one examines the complexity of animal and human behaviour, the world's cultural achievements and the more profound thinking associated with the major religions, wisdom-traditions and philosophies of the world, then it is very parsimonious indeed to put all of this down to some unprompted evolutionary "accident" as the advocates of biological primacy postulate. Even at the animal level the intricacies of mimicry, caring, nurturing and mating behaviour are suspiciously more complex and purposeful than can readily be accounted for by natural selection and "genetic drift". Simply throwing in the "solution" of the passage of time does not solve this dilemma. Who really believes that had monkeys type-writers and interminable time, they would ever accidentally produce anything resembling the works of Shakespeare, Proust, Dante or Goethe?

The current reductionistic trend towards bio-medical materialism, with its over-reliance on bio-technology and pharmacotherapy, is at risk of losing sight of the psycho-social and spiritual aspects of what it is to be human. I gave the example of the Darwinian view of evolution to highlight that those theories which focus exclusively on the biological domain are simplifying the enormous complexities involved.

Objections may also be raised to the alternative suggestion that "universal mind" somehow "causes" matter, i.e. that matter is mind-made. Another view is that mind and matter co-evolve and are not separate entities, but rather manifestations of the same phenomenon *at different levels of abstraction*. In other words, the dualistic view of linear causality, as in biological determinism, whereby matter "causes" mind (or vice versa), is usefully replaced by the notion of "linguistic parallelism" in which psyche and soma (e.g. mind and brain) are perceived as polymorphic manifestations at different levels of abstraction (Hogan, 1995). Here, by way of a crude analogy, we can think, metaphorically, of water molecules existing polymorphically in solid, liquid and gaseous forms. Notions of simple linear causality, with its attendant concern with one-way primary causes, are no longer seen to be useful. Circular causality, which can also include the concept of an "ultima ratio" (a direction or an ultimate raison d'être), is probably a more useful way to conceive of evolution. With this view, aetiology, the push of the past, is systemically balanced by teleology - the pull of the future.

Looking at causality as being circular, rather than linear, has implications for therapy praxis. If the relationship between mind and body is in *both* directions then so is the genesis of illness and its treatment (see DelMonte, 1996a). Western psychologists tend to give priority to the mind - as exemplified by the practice of psychotherapy (especially cognitive therapy), which is largely a "mind over matter" approach using prescribed verbalisation. Other approaches, mostly but not exclusively Eastern, focus more on silence and the stillness of meditation and how the trained body in turn affects the mind, as in Yoga, Aikido and Qi-gong (see DelMonte, 1995, and my next presentation, DelMonte, 1996b). Systemic-constructivist psychotherapists see the relationship between mind and body - as well as that between minds - as circular. Here they may agree with Buddhists who also hold the view that, ultimately, "personal mind", although narcissistically seductive, is no more than a window (usually with its blinds closed!) onto universal mind. Moreover, personal mind is subjected to unconscious forces, as well as to systemic pressures and becomes increasingly irrelevant as we inescapably approach death!

When it comes to psycho-analysts it can be argued that many key authors, like Melanie Klein and even Sigmund Freud, took a biological and aetiological approach in which the "push" of innate instincts, drives and unconscious phantasy play a determining role (see Fisher & Greenberg, 1996). Jung's view, like I have already suggested, was more teleological and thus juxtapositioned to that of Freud's in that he considered the *ultima ratio* (i.e. the pull) of universal mind, of archetypes and of the collective unconscious in shaping the human condition. Here, "universal mind" uses the organic domain to express itself - just like thoughts "use" thinkers to think them (Bion, 1970)!

I think that those stances to health which carry the message that life (evolution) has no meaning are doing a dis-service to patients who are trying to make sense of their experiences but nevertheless feel stuck and unable to do so. Could it be that one factor in the recent rise in suicides in the Western world is that young people are increasingly being raised in a reductionistic scientific culture which conveys the message that our existence is a meaningless bio-chemical "accident". Do some therapists, albeit unwittingly, further contribute to this problem by conveying a similar message?

References

1. Bion, W.R. (1970). *Attention and Interpretation*, Tavistock, London.
2. DelMonte, M.M. (1995). Silence and emptiness in the service of healing: Lessons from meditation. *British Journal of Psychotherapy*, 11(3), 368-378.
3. DelMonte, M.M. (1996a). Systems theory and psychotherapy: A constructivist perspective. In. M.G.T. Kwee and T.L. Holdstock (Eds), *Western and Buddhist Psychology: Clinical Perspectives*, Eburon, Delft, pp.269-293.
4. DelMonte, M.M. (1996b). The embodied mind, the talking cure and the silence of meditation. Paper also read at the International Congress of Psychotherapy, Satellite Conference, Body over mind or mind over body: Does it matter? Manoir D'Youville, Chateauquay, Montreal, Canada, August.
5. Fisher, S. & Greenberg, R.P. (1996). *Freud Scientifically Reappraised*. John Wiley & Sons, New York.
6. Hogan, C.C. (1995). *Psychosomatics, Psychoanalysis and Inflammatory Disease of the Colon*; International Universities Press, Madison, Connecticut.
7. Jung, C. (1958). Psychological commentary on the Tibetan book of the great liberation. In. *Psychology and Religion, Vol.2, Collected Works*, Pantheon Books, New York.
8. Reville, W. (1996). Science Today, *The Irish Times*, 9th September, Dublin.
9. Teilhard de Chardin, P. (1965). *The Phenomenon of Man*, Fontana, London.

DOES IT MATTER IF THE MEDITATOR DOES NOT MIND? - ON CONSCIOUSNESS AND AWARENESS OF THE BASIC I.D.

Maurits G.T. Kwee, Ph.D.
Head of the Inpatient Department of Behavioural Psychotherapy, Psychiatric Centre Joris, Delft, the Netherlands

Abstract

DOES IT MATTER IF THE MEDITATOR DOES NOT MIND? This question can only be well understood when placed in the context of the title of the symposium it belongs to, namely "Body over mind, or mind over body: Does it matter?". Obviously the title of this presentation is a rhetorical one, thus the answer is already included in the question. It does, however, matter to the clinical scientist who tries to transcend dualistic notions and uses for that purpose the semantics of "bodymind". The axioms of wholeness, consciousness and awareness are highlighted, and sophisticated studies that possess a power to reveal some of the hidden processes are reviewed. Psychoneuroimmunology promises to provide the microscopic proof for wholeness and the beneficial effects of self-awareness. But whether there exists a proclivity of mind over body, that the mentalists among us would like to see, will likely remain unknown. In the meantime a working hypothesis that gives the two equal weight provides a scientific model based on homeostasis and systemic thinking.
A multimodal systems view that bears in mind the *BASIC I.D.* (Behaviour, Affect, Sensation, Imagery, Cognition, Interpersonal relations and Drugs related biological issues) contends that emotions form the prototype of "mindbody" phenomena. Affect, feelings, and moods can be traced back to a hypothesised number of seven basic emotions. The meditator's "spiritual" path is to traverse depression, fear, anger, sadness, joy and love so as to arrive at serenity or silence. At this point all questions are recognised as illusory and finally dissolve. Meditation, e.g. Zen, promises to be one of the useful prophylactic means in the prevention of emotional disturbance, such as depression and all its biopsychosocial ramifications. The author further submits that Zen is a helpful discipline to maintain or improve the mental health of mental health professionals.

Chui, the draftsman
Is able to draw
More perfect circles freehand
Than with a compass
His fingers brought forth
Spontaneous forms from nowhere

His mind was meanwhile free
And without concern

No drives, no compulsions,
No needs, no atractions,
Then his affairs are under control
He is a free man

Chuang Tze
4th century B.C.

Credo Quia Absurdum
(I believe because it's absurd)

Instantaneous configurational changes in receptors of neurons during neurotransmission of neuropeptides give rise to the speculation that they posess "wave" and "particle" like characteristics (Pert, 1987). This notion suggests an analogy between exclusively mind *versus* body or brain theories and wave *versus* particle theories of subatomic physics. Quantum physics entails the renunciation of the classical (Newtonian) idea of causality. One of its tenets is based on observations in light radiation experiments that it was impossible to localise waves or particles in space and time with precision. Under one set of experimental conditions spontaneous and induced emission of radiation is explicable only by quantised particles. Under another set the interference patterns are explicable only by wave theory. Electrons, neurons, and photons can take the form of particles and waves in an unpredictable manner. The observer is not able to measure because observation itself changes physical reality. This dated fact is known nowadays as Heisenberg's uncertainty principle. The participant observer and the observed matter relate like a subject and an object that are interdependent and inseparable. It seems that there is no such thing as a tangible or complete measurable reality on a molecular or sub-atomic level of knowing and existence. These findings have resulted ultimately in introducing the concepts of wholeness, consciousness, and awareness by some phycisists (Capra, 1977; Zukav, 1979).

What can we (clinical) psychologists and other mental health workers learn from this experience? Most importantly the lesson that we should not try to imitate physical science, but to acknowledge the nature of human consciousness as the only rational base wherupon to build a viable science of psychology. However, most studies of body-mind relationships follow the prevailing framework of Cartesian (17th. century) metaphysical dualism. Within this paradigm mind and body are considered to be separate substances that function in parallel. Such a framework leads necessarily to mechanistic and reductionistic notions.

Reductionism is the philosophy that events can be understood by reducing them to their component parts on an increasingly smaller scale. Thus, if a problem can be described biologically the treatment of choice should be accordingly biological. The reduction of depressive disorders to certain neurotransmitter deficits and the reasoning that these can sufficiently be treated by merely prescribing a serotonin reuptake inhibitor is a recent example. However effective such an intervention might be, affective experiences are not likely to be grasped in an exclusively mechanistic way.

The antithesis of Cartesian dualism can be found in Spinozian monism. According to Spinoza (1632-1677), the contradictions in the universe are manifestations of one ultimate spiritual principle. This entails the philosophy that body-and-mind form an indivisable whole. The description of bodily processes and mind processes are just two different ways of expression that refer to one and the same divine substance (comparable to "soul" or consciousness). However absurd it may sound, those processes are supposed here to be logically complementary, analogous to the wave and particle theories that do not contradict but complement each other (Capra, 1977; Zukav, 1979).

Consequently, conceptual statements about the mental field of knowledge are not reducible to (nor deducible from) conceptual statements about the physical field of knowledge. No discovery in brain chemistry will likely ever lead to the reduction or explanation of consciousness. Human beings are material entities posessing inherently the faculty of consciousness that is necessary for perception and for acquiring any knowledge. To restate the essence of the present issue: Psychological terminology and biological terminology have the same indivisable concrete referents in nature, for instance depression, but different pathways of abstraction and networks of concepts. Each is equally true and valid within its own linguistic frame of reference and methodology. This purview concurs with "organic unity theory" (Goodman, 1991; Gomes, 1995).

Axioms and Essential Concepts

The purpose of this chapter is to stimulate the reader's interest in how to raise consciousness and develop awareness of the essential wholeness of one's being including the diversity of its manifestations on the surface. The target group: All mental health workers who (a) have discovered that neither learning therapy, nor supervision nor intervision are adequate measures to stimulate their own mental health, and (b) are ready to work on their own personal growth by (Zen) meditation, i.e. through the development of (self-)awareness (Kwee, 1996a). Before proceeding any further we need to define the axioms and essential terms employed throughout this chapter.

The axioms of wholeness, consciousness, and awareness are essential for a meditative discipline like Zen. These concepts are not proven but are the basis for all proof. They are irreducible facts of reality, self-evident to perception, and form the basis of all further knowledge. *Consciousness* is defined here as an emerging property and function of mind-body-as-an-indivisable-whole that does not possess the same attributes like inanimate matter. According to James (1903) it is the most mysterious thing in the world, that in fact is no actual thing but a non-entity (Natsoulas, 1978). Consciousness flows in a stream, that like a river springs from a source of bodymind. Its meaning comes closest to "soul", that is part of nature's eternal vital life energy. (In fact soul is the pejorative term for consciousness that was used by the early behaviourists.) Consciousness that exerts functional action will be called *awareness*. Consciousness denotes that one is aware of body/mind existence in general and all its manifestations in particular. Aware-

ness is distinguished by neutral attention that is paid to something (anything) and is a prerequisite for any human experience. Awareness includes self-awareness, a form of self-reflexiveness that is unique to human beings (e.g. to think that one thinks that one thinks, etc.). There are at least two levels of awareness: the perceptual-sensory level, involving exteroception and interoception, and the conceptual-rational level.
Consciousness makes self-awareness and thus introspection possible. Introspection is an appropriate method to come into contact with mind/body and to scrutinise one's own mental processes. Verbal reports can accurately reflect what a person is experiencing (cf. Davison, Navarre, & Vogel, 1995). Concentrated but nonjudgmental attention directed or guided to specific manifestations of body/mind, e.g. one's breathing, is called meditation. In my version of Zen the *meditator* is aware or mindful of (or better, witnesses) the contents and the processes of her or his particular Behaviours, Affects, Sensations, Images, Cognitions, Interpersonal relationships and biological changes (called Drugs for euphonic reasons). These modalities of the mind/body can be subsumed under the mnemonic acronym *BASICI.D.* (A. Lazarus, 1989), to be outlined further in one of the next paragraphs. My special interest in this chapter is to highlight the self-awareness of affective experience, the *tertium quid* (the third factor between two opposites), in order to better understand the nature of man as a physical-psychological-and-spiritual being.
The first measure is to become aware of the organic unity of body-and-mind by watching our rational-conceptual semantics. Terms like: matter-spirit, biological-psychological, physical-mental, body-and-mind separate components that are inherently inseparable in the nature of the things. The division exists only in our conceptualisation of perceived reality and the language that we use. The proposition that there is no mind without body and no body without mind like two sides of one coin should be reflected in our word usage. According to Korzybski (1933), the best way to use semantically correct words is to design a spelling that correctly reflects its concrete referents, like a map that is structurally similar to the territory it represents. In order to prevent one from getting lost in the process of abstraction, when using words about words about words, etc., he recommends amongst others to stop using the above mentioned elementalistic terms in isolation and to use instead a hyphen in between (e.g. body-mind) in writing as well as in thinking.
In my view a hyphen still reflects an elementalistic division. A far better semantic solution is to write each pair as one word and between quotation marks. Thus as "matterspirit" (or "spiritmatter"), "physicalmental" (or "mentalphysical"), "biopsychological" (or "psychobiological"), "*bodymind*" (or "*mindbody*"), etc., each pair of words to be used interchangeably. Note that I did not use the term psychosomatic because its semantic meaning in the scientific literature still implies a dualistic connotation of parallelism and interactionism (Graham, 1967).
How does the whole of the "bodymind" or the *BASICI.D.*, consciousness and awareness relate to each other? I see consciousness as an emergent property and function of "mindbody" on top of the triangle (cf. Sperry, 1969). The "bodymind" is an irreducible axiom with physical characteristics - particularly a complex spatiotemporal neural configuration of one billion cells - out of which consciousness, a pure mental phenomenon without physical characteristics, arises. Consciousness is more than the sum of its indivisable "parts" that are wrongly separated in body and mind (Globus, 1973). Awareness

as an exerting function of consciousness has a regulating effect on the "mindbody" via its concrete manifestations. It is my contention that awareness should be accorded primacy in the exertion of control over the *BASICI.D.* as the present operationalisation of the "bodymind".

A Matter of Consciousness

Although I was brought up professionally under the influence of Pavlov, Watson, and Skinner, my clinical work of the past 23 years makes it necessary to discard the basic tenets of behaviourism. I agree with Locke (1995) who contends:

At root behaviorism represents a form of mysticism - not religious mysticism but materialist mysticism; it reflects an unlimited faith in the power of the materialistic approach to understanding man ... behaviorism is profoundly nonobjective. It was able to rob man of freedom and dignity only by denying the self-evident fact of his mind. Psychology should not apologize for the fact that its subject matter does not consist of inanimate matter. It should start by honestly acknowledging what man is. In short, it is time we took consciousness seriously (p. 272).

Although consciousness and awareness could not exist without a certain type of brain, the particular way in which the "mindbody" makes consciousness possible and how awareness causes action is unknown. This does not mean that consciousness and awareness belong to the ineffable. It just means that these are the natural attributes of certain living entities. The attention that is paid during awareness is volitional. This entails the ability to regulate one's own acting. It involves free will or the choice to focus one's awareness on whatever sense perception or thought. That is a form of causality. The choice to perceive and think or not to perceive and not think is not uncaused, it is self-caused (Binswanger, 1991).

Consciousness and "bodymind" are also self-caused, that is: being cause *and* effect at the same time. Their relationship calls for a circular instead of linear causality. Thus, the state and condition of "mindbody" influence the quality of consciousness as the product of emergence that in its turn influences the quality of the self-awareness exerted on the "bodymind" (the *BASICI.D.*). In my clinical practice I regularly meet clients who repress their emotions to such an extent that they experience a dualism of "mindbody," a kind of splitting that might be proven if we were able to measure it. They emote less and might become numb in the end, having lost their sensory ability of touch. It can be safely speculated that emotional repression leads to a decreased health quality of "bodymind," like for instance in depression, and that this condition lowers the client's level of consciousness and awareness. In the remaining text I shall restrict the meaning of conscious awareness to emotional experiences.

Systems theory helps to develop the present theory of consciousness (Von Bertalanffy, 1968; Miller, 1978; Engel, 1977; Schwarz, 1984; Kwee & A. Lazarus, 1986; Kwee, 1996). The emergence of consciousness can either be in an "upward" (progressive) or in a "downward" (regressive) direction. The first leads to order (negentropy) and the second to chaos (entropy). The baseline is a neutral affective steady state that oscillates between reasonable boundaries. This state can change towards either a positive (higher) or a negative (lower) level of consciousness. This systemic conceptualisation leaves open the possibility of ascending bottom-up from the lower levels to the higher levels of consciousness. It is assumed that growth of consciousness is facilitated and takes place through a learning process of (self-)awareness regarding the meaning(fulness) of the negative affect that one experiences in life. "Normal" conscious affective experience is a volatile process that swings up and down around the baseline. This ranges between the familiar experiences of joy and sadness, love and anger, serenity and fear, as well as at some lower intensities of depression.

Consciousness and Affect

The notion of different levels of conscious experience implies that there can also be nonconscious processes (not to be confused with the psychodynamic unconscious) that are worth mentioning in this respect. Nonconscious phenomena especially of a repressive nature have to be assumed for all psychological theories (Shevrin & Dickman, 1980). Defensive reactions like regression, projection, displacement, disowning, splitting, and denial ward off negative affective experience. It is hypothesised that these self-deceptive manoeuvres contribute significantly to the development of lower levels of consciousness and affective awareness that might ultimately lead to the lowest level of a depressive state.

Depression starts as a "downward" submergent property of "bodymind" transversing lower levels of affective consciousness (basically sadness, anger and fear) in a spiralling process. The arrows upwards denote the possibility of creating order out of chaos through awareness of the *meaning* of one's depression. However, the clinician encounters mostly depressive states that are closely connected to and interact with "mindbody" in a circular causal manner in such a way that effect becomes cause and cause becomes effect. The long-term result could be a clinical detrimental affective condition wherein the individual's integrity - defined as "bodymind" plus consciousness - becomes disrupted and finally falls apart. Indeed there is convincing evidence suggesting that depressive disorders are associated with increased mortality which are not due to an excess of suicide (e.g. Elliot & Eisdorfer, 1982; O'Brien & Ames, 1994).
How does one conceive the "mindbody" question in the case of clinical depression? Modern clinical psychology and biological psychiatry offer two different linguistic approaches to the same aberrant condition. It can be formulated either in physical terms of neurotransmission or in mental terms of dysfunctional cognitions. One should be aware that each of these conceptualisations is reductionistic. The reduction of a dysfunctional or irrational idea to the statement that neuron A has sent an electrical impulse to neuron B just does not make sense. Therefore, one must indeed be *constantly* aware that this differentiation is due to an artificial separation of "mindbody", rather than in an embededness in its very nature that conceives oneness in different qualities. Thus, although it can be described in the terminological networks of either biology or

psychology, depression in all its varieties is considered to be a "bodymind" condition. According to "organic unity theory":

Neurotic conditions and personality disorders are no less biological than are schizophrenia and mood disorders, and the latter are no less biological than the former. Perhaps schizophrenia and mood disorders are considered to be more biological because they have more known features that readily fit the schemata for biological data and they have been more clearly defined in intersubjectively confirmable terms...The argument that genetic evidence for hereditary transmission indicates a biological rather than a psychological disorder is predicated on the erroneous equation of genetic with biological and of psychological with environmental, as well as the erroneous dichotomization of the biological and the psychological. What is inherited are *genetically encoded predispositions to the development of events and processes... Which may be referred to by and understood in terms of both biological and psychological concepts* (Goodman, 1991, p. 560; italics added).

It is a matter of awareness to adapt a nondualistic philosophy that considers neurosis no less biological than psychosis, and psychosis no less psychological than neurosis. This purview makes pharmacotherapy also a psychological treatment and psychotherapy also a biological treatment. Psycho-neuroimmunological research is beginning to provide the evidence for this contention as will be outlined later on. Let us first operationalise the "mindbody" by going into its manifestations, the *BASIC I.D.*

Multimodal Firing Orders

Once we have imbibed a "bodymind" wholistic awareness, we should exert it throughout our reasoning with all its ramifications. The multimodal approach is mindful of the *BASIC I.D.* (A. Lazarus, 1989). (A whole that is more than the sum of its modalities). Each modality refers to a "mindbody" function that, based on introspection and observation, can be classified as follows:

*B*ehaviour: The awareness of what one does, one's deeds, actions, gestures or habits that are observable.
*A*ffect: The awareness of one's inner feelings, moods, and especially emotions (primary) or blends of emotions (secondary, tertiary, etc).
*S*ensation: The awareness of sensory experiences (perceptions) like: seeing, hearing, smelling, tasting, and touching.
*I*magery: The awareness of what one sees in the mind's eye, mental pictures, fantasies, daydreams, visualisations (e.g. self-image).
*C*ognition: The awareness of one's analytical thinking, reasoning, or planning that can be rational (relative) or irrational (absolute).
*I*nterpersonal: The awareness of one's interactions with others relations and the tendency to gravitate toward one person or a group of people.
*D*rugs or biology: The awareness of bodily signals and physiology connected to the experience of whole body health, illness or disease.

On a macroscopic level each modality of the *BASIC I.D.* represents a major subject in psychology as an empirical science. The rationale to make this distinction on the microscopic or individual level lies in the fact that the content of awareness can be differentiated accordingly. The various modalities appear in the individual's awareness in a time sequence. Just like a diamond that reflects light on its facets one at a time, modalities shine in our awareness in firing orders. From a meditator's (but also clinician's) point of view, *Affect* is the most important modality. Its nature can be better understood when we realise that *Affect* always appears in awareness amidst other modalities. In theory there exist 5040 (7!) possible firing orders of the *BASIC I.D.* A sequential description of affective or emotional experience finds close connection with conceptualisations in the literature of emotion theories. The role of emotion as a bridging function *par excellence* in "mindbody" matters cannot be overemphasised (Kwee, 1996b).

Three major traditions can be distinguished in the theorising on emotions. Each can be described in terms of the person's awareness of firing orders. The *first* is *SBAC/I*: John Doe perceives a bear (*S*), emits a behaviour, runs (*B*), feels fear (*A*), and finally thinks (*C/I*). This line of inquiry began with Charles Darwin who claims that emotion serves a psychoevolutionary goal (Plutchik, 1995). The *second* is *SC/IBA*: John Doe sees a bear (*S*), assesses danger immediately (*C/I*), trembles and runs (*B*), and finally emotes fear (*A*). This position of emotional awareness is known as the James-Lange theory. William James included interpretation in perception and identified not the instrumental action but the autonomic excitation as being the emotion. Thus the simplified version "one is sad because one cries" is inaccurate (Ellsworth, 1994). The *third* is *SC/IAB*: John Doe perceives a bear (*S*), infers/imagines danger (*C/I*), experiences (the bodily changes of) fear (*A*), and activates flight (*B*). This firing order of awareness, originally proposed by Walter Cannon (and Bard), is nowadays widely applied in the cognitive behavioural therapy framework (R. Lazarus, 1991; A. Lazarus, & C. Lazarus, 1990; Beck, 1976; Ellis, 1995).

The awareness of a firing order during an emotional episode is a momentary reflection on an ongoing flux. The stream of consciousness is arrested for a moment - like in taking a photograph - in order to be able to study a fragment of the process. There can be as many emotional theories as known firing orders. Being aware of firing orders as fluid and flexible processes makes theorising in circular causal loops possible. Such loops allow us to theorise further about different entries, exits and regulation by feedback and feedforward mechanisms (Kwee & A. Lazarus, 1986).

The awareness of firing orders has a special impact on the clinician who needs a strategy for diminishing some of the guesswork in choosing an appropriate technique. A. Lazarus (1989) innovated a procedure called *tracking* the firing order. This refers to the observation of people's awareness that many usually follow a preferred and therefore somewhat predictable sequence. For example, some have the awareness of a *SICA*sequence (*S*ensation, *I*magery, *C*ognition, *A*ffect), whereas others have a *CISA*-sequence (*C*ognition, *I*magery, *S*ensation, *A*ffect). Tracking the firing order helps to calibrate the rightness of fit of the proposed technique. Which is the preferred relaxation technique in our example? In the former instance (*SICA*) sensory techniques such as biofeedback-assisted or unassisted muscle relaxation, meditation, diaphragmatic breathing or other low-arousal techniques may be expected to be effective. But in the second instance (*CISA*) the application of cognitive and imagery techniques would be expected to yield effective results, because these would address relevant triggers (A. Lazarus & Mayne, 1980).

These clinical impressions have found some empirical support. "Behavioural reactors" responded relatively better to social skills training or exposure *in vivo* and "physical reactors" to relaxation training, whereas "cognitive reactors" did well with cognitive interventions. Consonant techniques appear to be effective in 80% of the cases being studied (Schwarz, Davison, & Goleman, 1978; Öst, Jerremalm, & Johansson, 1981; Öst, Johansson, & Jerremalm, 1982; Michelson, 1986). However, it seems that the awareness of firing orders of emotional episodes is not enough for comprehending what the quality of a specific emotion is. For that purpose we have to turn to the content of each of our emotional experiences and attend to the question: Which basic emotions can one be aware of?

The Varieties of Basic Emotions

Whereas in the previous paragraph *Affect* has been scrutinised in the context of the *BASIC I.D.*, here *Affect* will be analysed into its basic components. At this juncture it is necessary to be coherent and precise about the terms *Affect* and emotion that have been employed interchangeably in the foregoing sections. *Affect* is defined here as a concept that is more general than emotion. The latter is defined as a concept that is relatively more specific and restricted. Thus *Affect* includes emotion, but not all affective conditions have the intensity of an emotion (Clore, Ortony, & Foss, 1987). The cardinal question is: What constitutes a basic emotion? The awareness of a basic or primary emotion covers experiences that range from silence to strongly "herenow" deeply felt inner moving qualities. The experience of relatively weaker and more superficial states is called secondary (e.g. moods) or tertiary (e.g. feelings) emotions. A feeling can be a sensory experience but also an affective state that is less intense than a mood. The weaker the experienced state, the more awareness of contamination by the other modalities. The stronger the experienced state, the less awareness of involvement of other modalities.

The levels of emotional experience that one can be aware of is composed of two categories of three classes each. A class is centered around the experience of a basic emotion that was differentiated previously on theoretical grounds (Kwee, 1996). In addition to the description given before, an emotion is considered basic if it is *a universal experience, denoted by a term that is semantically unanalysable; furthermore the emotion is understood without having to appeal to any other feeling* (Johnson-Laird & Oatley, 1992). The awareness of higher levels of consciousness is optimal when the basic emotions of joy, love and serenity are experienced, whereas lower levels are at stake in case of sadness, anger, and fear. Prolonged experience of these negative emotions may result in clinical depression, a detrimental state characterised by a minimal level of awareness. Silence is also experienced during this state. However, this is a silence of a graveyard which is of another kind than salubrious silence as when oneness with nature is experienced. The latter sort of silence also marks the arrested or quiet state of non-emotion out of which all emotions (from Latin *emovere*: to move out or to stir up) emanate. Hence, silence and depression - as a beginning (order, negentropy) and end state (chaos, entropy) - are placed in opposite positions to indicate their complementary functions.

Awareness of different levels of emotional experience implies a labelling process of searching and finding a specific name for a specific basic emotion. This process of naming presupposes an awareness of the emotion and related cognitions such as lexical knowledge. Once a word is correctly found and identified with an emotion, mastery can be achieved over some emotional disturbances associated with alexithymia or dislexithymia. Both positively and negatively felt emotions can be functional and disfunctional.

Emotional Self-Awareness

The regressive emotions - sadness, anger, and fear - are functional whenever there is cognitive awareness of a natural connection between an event and the emotion. Thus in fear one is aware of a threat to attain a goal, in anger of a frustration in reaching a goal, and in sadness of some loss of a goal. These emotions are disfunctional when its appearance is so frequent and intense that a clinical disorder may be appropriately diagnosed. Panic, rage, or distress are usually disfunctional and overly repressed in many cases. The result of truncating one's awareness is that the person will report symptoms of pathology sooner or later.

The progressive emotions - joy, love, and serenity - posess healthy concomitants (see Kwee, 1996b) and are mostly functional. Some of their manifestation can be marked off distinctively as disfunctional, e.g. inadequate laughing, sexual aberrations, or apathetic escapism. Intense sadness and joy make people melt. Both are humid experiences. In joy there is an awareness of a progression towards a goal, in love of a merging with a goal, and in serenity the person experiences self-contentment while metaphorically there are no goals left.

Love heals, but the practice of love is one of the most difficult forms of art that exists. It is especially necessary, in my opinion, for clinicians to communicate the appropriate professional variety of love - compassion - to their clients. I have discovered that teasing the client playfully according to the wise old German saying "Wass sich liebt, dass neckt sich" (teasing is a way of loving) is a fruitful manner of establishing rapport during treatment. It is unnecessary to say that one should never belittle or offend the client in any way. Teasing empathically leads to an opening up of the client who comes out, at last, of her or his emotional shell. In most cases a greater sense of trust and understanding will paradoxically be achieved on the part of the client.

The basic emotions that I propose follow the ladder of consciousness. This covers a spectrum that varies from the lower levels (depression, fear, anger and sadness) to the higher levels (joy, love, serenity and silence). Perhaps silence is the least understood state of consciousness because it requires some openness to spirituality to appreciate the value of such an experience which is usually considered unscientific. James (1903) called it an "oceanic feeling", but it might also be called enlightenment, satori, Buddha-state, nirvana, Tao, or Christ-consciousness. These terms are impossible to explain further in words, hence the best name is silence (Kwee, 1990b).

What can help to distinguish levels of emotional awareness in a clinical or training situation is the ability to classify an affective term under one of the basic emotions. In such a way the therapist or trainer can develop a list that helps to identify families of basic emotions. Each family consists of words signifying the same basic emotional colour in different hues. No doubt there will be some overlap within the same basic colour and in-between the basic colours, but the principle of basic emotions remains intact.

Table 1. Clinical guide for differentiating levels of emotional awareness

Depression	Fear	Anger	Sadness	Joy	Love	Serenity	Silence
blues	worry	annoyance	pity	amused	tender-	relaxed	
dejection	apprehens-	contempt	sorrow	glad	ness	trustful	
dysphoria	ion	hostility	distress	happy	fondness	faithful	
down-	anguish	animosity	grief	good	intimacy	thankful	
hearted-	anxiety	fury	afflict-	hu-	compass-	safe	
ness	fright	rage	ion	mour	ion	secure	
despond-	horror	amok	agony	de-	in-	satisfied	
ency	terror	resent-	mourning	lighted	fatuation	peaceful	
low	panic	ment	hurt	euphoric	eroticism	etc	
spirits	etc...	etc...	etc...	manic	passion		
melancho-			content	affection			
lia				etc.	etc.	dysthymia	etc.

Table 1 is an illustration of such a list. The affective lexicon might consist of 4000 English words. However, not all of them refer to emotional states. For instance, acceptance, anticipation, disgust and surprise, which are all distinguished by Plutchik (1994) as basic emotions, are discarded as such from a multimodal point of view. Using the *BASIC I.D.* as a filter, acceptance and anticipation are identified as *C*ognitions, whilst disgust and surprise are perceptions(*S*). Other terms are relatively less emotional and more *B*ehavioural (e.g. willful), *A*ffective (e.g. affectionate), *S*ensory (e.g. pain), *I*maginative (e.g. pissed-off), *C*ognitive (e.g. guilt), *I*nterpersonal (e.g. unattractive), or physiological (*D.*) (e.g. perplexed). It is recommended also to be aware of affective terms that might be composed by a blend of emotions. For instance, the *I*mage "heartbroken" may refer to sadness and depression, the *C*ognition "guilt" to fear and sadness, the *A*ffect "lonely" to depression and fear, etc.

The correlation between negatively felt emotions and lowered levels of awareness deserves to be noticed. The clinical observation that emotional disturbance is accompanied by a narrowing of attention has lead to the idea that awareness decreases concomitantly. Attention becomes distracted and disarrayed in regressive emotional states as was confirmed convincingly by Gilligan and Bower (1984). They tested recall of either sad or happy material that was learned while the subjects were either in a sad or happy mood. Those who were more intensely happy remembered more of both the happy and sad material than those who were only mildly happy. But people who were more intensely sad remembered less of the material than people who were only mildly sad. It might be expected that highly intense negative emotions in general interfere with attentional processes of recall, retention, and thus with consciousness and self-awareness.

Depression, Repression and Suppression

Just like the mechanism of awareness is (neutral) attention, the mechanism of self-awareness is self-attention. It is proposed that neutral self-attention strenghtens the health condition of "bodymind" and is thus beneficial for one's *BASIC I.D.* Too little, but also too much attention to emotional experiences may result in pathology. The relationship between self-attentional processes and health seems to take the form of an inverted U-shaped function (Vaillant, 1986).

In this model depression is a function of excessive attention that is paid to one's negative emotions with injurious effects to health, e.g. a decrease in immunity (to be elaborated later). Giving undue attention to one's own emotional problems means that positive feedback processes are at work. Positive feedback adds (hence positive) so much information that the *BASIC I.D.* will either get blocked or explodes. In depression augmented attention is allocated to negative ideation of oneself, one's relationships, and one's future, to the point that "distancing" is indicated (Beck, 1976). The same mechanism of positive feedback is at stake in the case of repression, a consequence of which is that particular feelings are kept out of consciousness. To a certain extent everybody uses repression, but if it is used unduly it becomes defensiveness: An unhealthy habit of beguiling oneself. The essential feature of severe repression is the progressive lack of attention to one's own existing negative emotional feelings (e.g. sadness) and connected behaviours (e.g. crying). In such a way, defensive people disconnect their real emotional feelings from what they (falsely) report they have experienced. These processes affect the *BASIC I.D.*'s steady state in an unhealthy way.

A healthy way to deal with self-attention is flexibility instead of rigidity. The ability to be flexible in paying and shifting one's attention to something is called suppression (Vaillant, 1986). Suppression is an adaptive strategy of postponing the decision to pay attention to one's problematic experiences. Thus, the person decides in full awareness, for instance, to pay attention to fear, anger or sadness at a particular moment but not at other moments. This process works on the basis of negative feedback mechanisms. Incoming information in our awareness is subtracted (hence negative) leading to a regression to the mean, i.e. to a steady state of the *BASIC I.D.* The difference with repression and depression is clear. In repression the existence of a negatively felt emotion is denied. In suppression that existence is acknowledged but consciously kept out of awareness. The attention is shifted towards something else momentarily. In depression one suffers from the bulk of emotional problems that one attends to. In suppression one is aware of one's negative emotions. The healthy option is to alternate one's attention and be aware of one's own capabilities as well. According to longitudinal studies by Vaillant (1986), conducted with a group of almost 200 adult males, the most succesful and healthy among them had a lifestyle characterised by a frequent use of suppression.

A repressive coping style will lead the person into emotional problems that may result ultimately in depression and other aberrant conditions. Schwartz's (1984) disregulation theory states that repression (disattention) leads to disease and awareness (self-attention) leads to health. How can self-attentional processes be healthy? When a person attends to some aspect of the *BASIC I.D.* he or she alters it whether one is or is not aware of the changes that are taking place. (This proposition is similar to the Heisenbergian principle that was mentioned in the beginning of this paper). If a person neutrally attends to her or his body (biology or *D.* modality) this will be beneficial for the "bodymind", since in our theory the body is inherently connected with the mind. The benefit of this awareness process is that the quality of the "mindbody" will improve and that higher levels of consciousness will emerge. In its turn this amplifies awareness that positive emotional experiences, such as those due to caring or relaxation, have health promoting consequences.

People who apply relaxed affiliative self-care procedures seem to profit from these beneficial consequences. There exist a number of self-attentional procedures that are supposed to function on the basis of feedback mechanisms. All kinds of self-care practices may have these health implications, such as clothing, hair-dressing, wearing jewelry, using perfume, etc.

An ancient way to apply self-attention is meditation, a process of non-judgmental watching or observing. This is the exertion of awareness on the "bodymind" and all its possible manifestations of the *BASIC I.D.* For instance, by witnessing one's breathing respiration becomes slower, deeper, and more regular, which has a stabilising impact on other observable "mindbody" functions. Relaxed self-attention to one's heart rate and respiration have self-regulatory effects especially when the attention is augmented by "natural biofeedback" (e.g. sensing the air coming out of the nose and feeling one's pulse).

Is Psychotherapy a Biological Treatment?

Some changes in the *BASIC I.D.* take place beyond our awareness, especially those changes at the cellular level. Because these go unnoticed there is no immediate corrective feedback possible. However, knowledge derived from laboratory studies can serve as indirect feedback to sharpen our awareness of the existence of microscopic processes and to adjust our attentional strategies accordingly. Scientific progress in the field of psycho-neuroimmunology has provided a beginning for evidence of the "bodymind" as an indivisable organic unity. Psycho-neuroimmunology is the integrated study of behavioural-neural-endocrine-immune system interactions.

Psycho-neuroimmunology began with the discovery that the immune system is able to learn. Nearly two decades ago Robert Ader did classical conditioning experiments with rats by giving them an immunity inhibiting substance plus saccharine. After a few couplings saccharine alone could bring about the immuno-suppressive response. Moreover, nerve fibres were found in the spleen where they were not supposed to be located. The conclusion of these findings is trail-blazing. The central nervous system is connected with the immune system that hitherto was thought to be functioning autonomously.

The "mindbody" is interconnected and emotions play an important role in our health. The new field of psycho-neuroimmunology promises to offer a body of evidence that might support the notions on "mindbody" wholeness that I espouse here. Alas, the present state of the art is such that a direct causal link between affect, diminished immune function and disease has yet to be established (Ader, Cohen, & Felten, 1995).

Nevertheless, there are strong empirical indications that stressful experiences associated with a variety of negative emotions, particularly sadness due to bereavement and other losses like marital separation, modulate immune functions substantially (Bartrop, L. Lazarus, Luckhurst, Kiloh, & Penny, 1977; Glaser, Kiecolt-Glaser, Speicher, & Holiday, 1985; Irwin, Daniels, Smith, Bloom & Weiner, 1987). Furthermore, a meta-analysis reviewing studies on clinical *depression* and immunity up to 1991 revealed reliable effects (Herbert & Cohen, 1993). The immune alterations were measured by enumerative (numerical decreases in T, B, and NK cells) and functional (lymphocyte proliferative responses to mitogens and reduced NK cell activity) parameters. A recent meta-analytic review showed a linear relation between depressive affect and the indicators of cellular immunity (cf. Schleier, Keller, Bartlett, Eckholdt, & Delaney, 1996). The alterations were greater in both hospitalised and older subjects. With respect to the immuno-modulating effects of *anger* and *fear* only a few studies exists with slightly favourable results (Gerritsen, Heynen, Wiegant, Bermond, & Fryda, 1996; La Via, Munno, Lydiard, Workman, Hubbard, Michel, & Paulling, 1996). Methodological problems connected with the - difficult to control - deleterious effect on immunity of, for example, sleep, smoking, alcohol consumption, etc. hamper the design of sound studies (Surman, Williams, Sheehan, Strom, Jones, & Coleman, 1986; Wiedenfeld, O'Leary, Bandura, Brown, Levine, & Raska, 1990; Futterman, Kemeny, Shapiro, & Fahey, 1992).

Less evidence exists for immune alterations associated with explicit positive emotional states including humour and relaxation. Recently Kiecolt-Glaser and Glaser (1992) reviewed the immunological changes that have been associated with psychological interventions. Several studies are methodologically weak because of using only secretory immunoglobulin A (IgA) as the dependent variable (e.g. Dillon, Minchoff, & Baker, 1986; McClelland & Kirshnit, 1988). Relaxation seems to have a prophylactic value for NK cell activity and T helper lymphocyte percentages in medical students during examinations (Kiecolt-Glaser, Glaser, Strain, Stout, Tarr, Holliday, & Speicher, 1986) and is able to increase NK cell activity and bring about a decrease in antibody titers to Herpes Simplex Virus in a geriatric sample (Kiecolt-Glaser, Glaser, Williger, Stout, Messick, Sheppard, Ricker, Romisher, Briner, Bonnell, & Donnerberg, 1985). It is suggested that stress-reduction has a minimal impact on the immunity of young, healthy, and nondistressed individuals. Furthermore, it is not advisable to exceed normal levels, because more is not necessarily better. Conclusive evidence is lacking with regard to the effects of relaxation on immunity (Van Rood, 1990; Van Rood, Boogaards, Goulmy, & Van Houwelingen, 1993).

An intriguing line of psycho-neuroimmunological research has been initiated by Pennebaker and his co-workers (Pennebaker, 1993). They asked themselves whether stress can be put into words. The experimental procedure of "putting stress into words" typically consists of asking subjects to write about deeply emotional experiences - such as

the most traumatic experience of one's entire life - for three to four consecutive days during 15 to 20 minutes a day. Across several studies it was found that such a disclosure is quite powerful in bringing about meaningful results. The effects were substantiated by significant drops in a number of variables such as health centre or physician visits, fewer absentee days, improved liver enzyme function, enhanced and more efficient immune function (Pennebaker & Beall, 1986; Francis & Pennebaker, 1992; Greenberg & Stone, 1992; Pennebaker, Kiecolt-Glaser, & Glaser, 1988; Esterling, Antoni, Kumar, & Schneiderman, 1990). These changes could not be accounted for by a change in healthier lifestyle due to the writing nor by a difference in the topics of writing.
It is worthwile to delve into two of these experiments because they link the exertion of self-awareness by lifting, one's repression by writing about traumatic experiences. Pennebaker, Kiecolt-Glaser and Glaser (1988) assigned fifty undergraduates either to write about trivial events or traumatic experiences varying from leaving home to sexual abuse. Compared to control subjects the experimental group, who wrote about upsetting events, showed significantly higher lymphocyte responses to stimulation by two types of mitogens (PHA and Con A). Furthermore, subjects who previously held back their traumatic experiences had a better T cell proliferative response than subjects who had shared their traumatic experiences with others before. In another study (Petrie, Booth, Pennebaker, Davison, & Thomas, 1995) the focus is on the question whether emotional writing about traumas is able to influence subjects who tested negative for hepatitis B antibodies. As compared to a control group the experimental group showed significantly higher antibody levels against hepatitis B on follow-up at six months. This finding further supports the healthy effects of emotional expression.

Analyses of the writings indicate that the topics in the treatment condition vary and include relational disruption, leaving home, and physical or psychological abuse. Participants whose health variables increased most used significantly more negative emotion words (e.g. sad, hate, or guilt) and fewer positive emotion words (e.g. joy, happy, or peaceful) than those who did not change. The no-change subjects showed a tendency to use relatively more positive words over time. Negative emotion words bring about immediate though short-lived heightened skin conductance levels as measured by a computer keyboard. Positive emotion words were typically linked with instant drops in arousal levels. It seems that there is no gain without pain. Confronting upsetting experiences is beneficial on the long run. "Across the various studies, ratings and/or indices of negative and positive emotions were unrelated to the cognitive dimensions. Both emotional and cognitive factors independently predict improvements in health and changes in autonomic activity" (Pennebaker, 1993, p. 546).
Generally speaking, the results suggest that psychological treatment that puts emotional stress into words are also biological. It seems that biological changes reflect psychological aberrations in the emotional disorders. Psychotherapy should be considered a biological treatment because it also acts through biological mechanisms on biological problems. The fact that the language of psychology serves better than the language of biology (e.g. neurotransmitters, synapses, and brain structures) when discussing psychotherapy with clients does not obviate the expanded meaning given to the psychological terms by the hardwired data (cf. Eisenberg, 1995; Mohl, 1987). It is the task of

the clinical scientist to make her or his clients aware of these new findings in order to help them to adopt a healthy lifestyle.

Adopting a Meditative Livestyle

If one already lives an emotionally healthy life, for instance through practicing meditation like Zen, biological changes are less impressive (Delmonte, 1984, 1990). Then the benefits of meditation take place relatively more on the psychosocial levels (the *BASI-CI.* instead of the *D.*). Or the meditator will rather experience a spiritual quality in life by her or his practice. By meditation, and by the process of witnessing, one becomes aware of having a "soul," just like seeing and hearing can make one become aware of having eyes and ears.

Since its inception as a scientific discipline (clinical) psychology has concurrently become "de-souled" (Kwee & Holdstock, 1996). By taking consciousness and awareness into account a "soul-like" quality can be restored to the quest of human life. From a multimodal perspective the heightening of (self-)awareness is one of the main hypothesised mechanisms of change. When talking about (self-)awareness and (self-)attentional processes we touch the essence of meditation practice. The exertion of awareness, i.e. the voluntary deployment of attention, forms the heart of meditation. Mental health workers who want to maintain their own mental health or strive for growth are recommended to adopt a meditative lifestyle that is expected at least to help in preventing the practitioner from developing an emotional disorder.

That the formal practice of meditation can be an important prophylaxis has also been put forward recently by some cognitive-behavioural therapists (Teasdale, Segal, & Williams, 1995). In what they call ATC (Attentional Control Training) a combination of meditation and *cognitive restructuring* à la Tim Beck is proposed. Meditation is an attractive technique as a generic stress-reduction technique that can be learned while in a balanced state. Kabat-Zinn's (1990) well-documented Buddhist inspired mindfulness training provides the basis for a formal practice that consists of an eight weekly 2-hour group programme. During these sessions the participants sit quietly in an erect posture while attempting in a non-striving way to maintain attention on one's own breathing. When the attention wanders off the person re-directs the attention gently back to the "here-now" of the breath, thus creating a meta-state of distancing. Whenever attention is drifting away to thoughts, feelings, or any other stress-related experience one stays in the present moment accepting everything just as it is without trying to change it. A heightened state of awareness will be the result which is different from operating in an "automatic pilot" or mindless mode. The person feels joyous and experiences her or his daily activities as if returned from holidays. The prophylactic value, for instance with respect to depression, is that the person will discover any automatic depressogenic signs timely.

However, it might be possible that a meditative lifestyle is difficult to implement because of too much repression. In that case psychotherapy by *emotional restructuring* may be prescribed (Kwee, 1996b). This innovative technique is based on two basic principles, namely feeling identification and "owning" one's feelings. When one gets to know the word for an emotion that was repressed, one breaks the "magic spell" that was put on one that frequently resulted in agony and despair. The essence of emotional restructuring as a technique is to be able (a) to identify a term as an affective term by using the *BASIC I.D.* as a filter (e.g. laughing is a behaviour, joy is an emotion), (b) to rubricise each affective term that one might use under one of the seven categories of basic emotions (e.g. apprehension belongs to the family of fear). As was experimentally proven by Pennebaker and co-workers the use of negative or positive emotion words does matter for one's healing and health. It is important for someone not only to have a vocabulary of affective terms, but also to apply these terms while being aware of its psycho-neuroimmunological implications.

This procedure might be viewed in the context of what has been called emotional intelligence (Goleman, 1995), which operates in dealing with emotions of others and of one's own. The basis for this capacity is the capacity for self-awareness that may lead to the assessment of how and what one feels, as well as the adequate use of one's feelings. Thus, not a vague feeling of dissatisfaction, but the recognition that one feels anger or sadness and the ability to witness the emotion from some inner distance. Many affective experiences go unnoticed. Awareness and voluntary attention to what one feels seem to be an exception in daily life for most people. Concentration cannot be enforced. It is rather based on one's being interested in what one experiences. Only after an awakening of this interest will a start in training to adopt a meditative lifestyle be possible. Some characteristics of such a lifestyle are (a) emotional involvement in whatever one exerts one's awareness, (b) intrinsic motivation that guarantees one's commitment, (c) flexibility and creativity in solving stumbling blocks on the path, (d) enjoyment in training and practicing the new lifestyle, and (e) "the art of laziness," meaning to relax by allowing oneself to be lazy from time to time. Such a training may result in higher forms of consciousness and subsequent awareness exertion.

A state of expanded consciousness and heightened awareness is a phenomenon known as *flow* (Czikzentmihalyi, 1978). This state is the opposite of worrying or throbbing and might as well be called an "egoless state of being." The key elements of flow are "(a) the merging of action and awareness in sustained concentration on the task at hand, (b) the focussing of attention in pure involvement without concern for outcome, (c) self-forgetfulness with heightened awareness of the activity, (d) skills adequate to meet the environmental demand, and (e) clarity regarding situational cues and appropriate response" (Goleman, 1990, p. 29). Flow can be observed in athletes, musicians, check players, mountain climbers, scientists, artists, and even book-keepers. Sports people call flow "the zone" in which they can achieve effortlessly and during which they merge with their sport in a sort of ecstatic state. In a way, playful children who are focussed on their game are also in a state of flow. An illustrative anecdote concerns a surgeon who was one day performing a difficult operation. He was so absorbed in his task that he forgot everything that happened around him. Not only was he amazed to discover that "time flies," it was two hours later, but neither did he notice that part of the ceiling fell down during his performance.

Goleman (1990) interprets flow in terms of neurophysiology. It is not an ongoing state of arousal but rather a state of activation that can change and is tailored to fluctuating situational requirements. Above all flow concurs with the Zen meditator's mental state:

perceptional clarity, alertness, equanimity, pliancy, efficiency and skill in action. In conclusion, the flow state can be one of the benefits of a meditative lifestyle that contributes to the mental health worker's full functioning, health, and self-actualisation. In a flow state the "bodymind" is experienced as a nondualistic whole. Then, it does not matter that the meditator does not mind, whether it is mind over body or body over mind.

References

Ader, R., Cohen, N., & Felton, D. (1995). Psychoneuroimmunology: Interactions between the nervous system and the immune system. *The Lancet, 345,* 99-103.

Bartrop, R., Lazarus, L., Luckhurst, E., Kiloh, L.G., & Penny, R. (1977). Depressed lymphocyte function after bereavement. *The Lancet, 327,* 834-836.

Beck, A.T. (1976). *Cognitive Therapy and the Emotional Disorders.* New York: International Universities Press.

Binswanger, H. (1991). Volition as cognitive self-regulation. *Organisational Behavior and Human Decision Processes, 50,* 154-178.

Capra, F. (1977). *The Tao of Physics.* New York: Bantam.

Clore, G.L., Ortony, A., & Foss, M.A. (1987). The psychological foundations of the affective lexicon. *Journal of Personality and Social Psychology, 53,* 751-766.

Czikzentmihalyi, M. (1978). *Between Boredom and Anxiety.* San Fransisco: Josey-Bass.

Davison, G.C., Navarre, S.G., & Vogel, R.S. (1995). The articulated thoughts in simulated situations paradigm: A think-aloud approach to cognitive assessment. *Psychological Science, 4,* 29-33.

DelMonte, M.M. (1985). Biochemical indices asociated with meditation practice: A literature review. *Neuroscience & Biobehavioural Reviews, 9,* 557-561.

DelMonte, M.M. (1990). The revelance of meditation to clinical practice: an overview. *Applied Psychology: An International Review, 39,* 331-354.

De Vries, M.J.C. (1986). Crisis en transformatie. *Medisch Contact, 24,* 751-756.

Dillon, K.M., Minchoff, B., & Baker, K.H. (1985). Positive emotional states and enhancement of the immune system. *International Journal of Psychiatry and Medicine, 1,* 13-18.

Eisenberg, L. (1986). Mindlessness and brainlessness in psychiatry. *British Journal of Psychiatry, 148,* 497-508.

Eisenberg, L. (1995). The social construction of the human brain. *American Journal of Psychiatry, 152,* 1563-1575.

Elliot, G.R., & Eisdorfer, C. (1982). *Stress and Human Health.* New York: Springer.

Ellis, A. (1995). Fundamentals of rational emotive behaviour therapy for the 1990s. In W. Dryden (Ed.), *Rational Emotive Behaviour Therapy* (pp. 1-30). London: Sage.

Ellsworth, P.C. (1994). William James and emotion: Is a century of fame worth a century of misunderstanding? *Psychological Review, 101,* 222-229.

Engel, G.L. (1977). The need for a new medical model: A challenge for biomedicine. *Science, 196,* 129-135.

Esterling, B., Antoni, M., Kumar, M., & Schneiderman, N. (1990). Emotional repression, stress disclosure responses, and Epstein-Barr viral lapsid antigen titers. *Psychosomatic Medicine, 52,* 397-410.

Francis, M.E., & Pennebaker, J.W. (1992). Putting stress into words: The impact of writing on physiological, absentee, and self-reported emotional well-being measures. *American Journal of Health Promotion, 6,* 280-287.

Futterman, A.D., Kemeny, M.E., Shapiro, D., & Fahey, J.L. (1992). Immunological variability associated with experimentally-induced positive and negative affective states. *Psychological Medicine, 22,* 231-238.

Gerritsen, W., Heynen, C.J., Wiegant, V.M., Bermontd, B., & Fryda, N.H. (1996). Experimental social fear: Immunological hormonal and autonomic concomitants. *Psychomatic Medicine, 58,* 273-286.

Gilligan, S.G., & Bower, G.H. (1984). Cognitive consequences of emotional arousal. In C.E. Izard, J. Kagan, & R.B. Zajonc (Eds.), *Emotions, Cognition, and Behavior.* New York: Cambridge University Press.

Glaser, R., Kiecolt-Glaser, J.K., Speicher, C.E., & Holiday, J.E. (1977). Stress, loneliness, and changes in herpesvirus latency. *Journal of Behavioral Medicine, 8,* 249-260.

Globus, G.G. (1973). Consciousness and brain: I. The identity thesis. *Archives of General Psychiatry, 29,* 153-160.

Goleman, D. (1990). The psychology of meditation. In M.G.T. Kwee (Ed.), *Psychotherapy, Meditation, and Health* (pp. 19-35). London: East-West.

Goleman, D. (1995). *Emotional Intelligence.* New York: Bantam Books.

Gomes, G. (1995). Self-awareness and the mind-brain problem. *Philosophical Psychology, 8,* 155-165.

Goodman, A. (1991). Organic unity theory: The mind-body problem revisited. *American Journal of Psychiatry, 148,* 553-563.

Graham, D.T. (1967). Health, disease, and the mind-body problem: Linguistic parallelism. *Psychosomatic Medicine, 29,* 52-71.

Greenberg, M.A., & Stone, A.A. (1992). Writing about disclosed versus undisclosed traumas: Immediate and long-term effect on mood and health. *Journal of Personality and Social Psychology, 63,* 75-84.

Herbert, T.B., & Cohen, S. (1993). Depression and immunity: A meta-analytic review. *Psychological Bulletin, 113,* 472-486.

Irwin, M., Daniels, M., Smith, T.L., Bloom, E., & Weiner, H. (1987). Impaired natural killer cell activity during bereavement. *Brain, Behaviour, and Immunity, 1,* 98-104.

James, W. (1903). *The Varieties of Religious Experience.* New York: Longmans-Green.

Johnson-Laird, P.N., & Oatley, K. (1992). Basic emotions, rationality, and folk theory. In N.L. Stein & K. Oatley (Eds.), *Basic Emotions* (pp. 201-224). Hove, UK: Lawrence Erlbaum.

Kabatt-Zinn, J. (1990). *Full Catastrophe Living.* New York: Delacorte Press.

Kiecolt-Glaser, J.K., & Glaser, R. (1992). Psychoneuroimmunology: Can psychological interventions modulate immunity? *Journal of Consulting and Clinical Psychology, 60,* 569-575.

Kiecolt-Glaser, J.K., Glaser, R., & Strain, E., Stout, J., Tarr, K., Holliday, J., & Speicher, C. (1986). Modulation of cellular immunity in medical students. *Journal of Behavioral Medicine, 9,* 5-21.

Kiecolt-Glaser, J.K., Glaser, R., Williger, D., Stout, J., Messick, G., Sheppard, S., Ricker, D., Romisher, S., Briner, W., Bonnell, G., & Donnerberg, R. (1985). Psychosocial enhancement of immunocompetence in a geriatric population. *Health Psychology, 4,* 25-41.

Korzybski, A. (1933). *Science and Sanity.* Lakeville, CON: Institute of General Semantics.

Kwee, M.G.T. (1990a). Health psychology and meditation by genuine laughing and smiling. In M.G.T. Kwee (Ed.), *Psychotherapy, Meditation, and Health: A Cognitive-Behavioural Perspective* (pp. 289-306). London: East-West.

Kwee, M.G.T. (Ed.). (1990b). *Psychotherapy, Meditation, and Health: A Cognitive-Behavioural Perspective.* London: East-West.

Kwee, M.G.T. (1996a). Travelling in the footsteps of Hotei towards the 21st century. In M.G.T. Kwee, & T.L. Holdstock (Eds.), *Western and Buddhist Psychology: Clinical Perspectives* (pp. 175-214). Delft, the Netherlands: Eburon.

Kwee, M.G.T. (1996b). A multimodal systems view on psyche, affect, and the basic emotions. In M.G.T. Kwee, & T.L. Holdstock (Eds.), *Western and Buddhist Psychology: Clinical Perspectives* (pp. 221-268). Delft, the Netherlands: Eburon.

Kwee, M.G.T., & Holdstock. T.L. (Eds.). (1996). *Western and Buddhist Psychology: Clinical Perspectives.* Delft, the Netherlands: Eburon.

Kwee, M.G.T., & Lazarus, A.A. (1986). Multimodal therapy: The cognitive-behavioural tradition and beyond. In W. Dryden, & W.L. Golden (Eds.), *Cognitive-Behavioural Approaches to Therapy* (pp. 320-355). London: Harper & Row.

La Via, M.F., Munno, I, Lydiard, B, Workman, E.W., Hubbard, J.R., Michel, Y., & Paulling, E. (1996). The influence of stress intrusion on immunodepression in generalized anxiety disorder patients and controls. *Psychosomatic Medicine, 58,* 138-142.

Lazarus, A.A. (1989). *The Practice of Multimodal Therapy.* Baltimore, ML: Johns Hopkins University Press.

Lazarus, A.A., & Lazarus, C.N. (1990). Emotions: A multimodal perspective. In H. Plutchik, & H. Kellerman (Eds.), *Emotion: Theory, Research, and Experience* (pp. 195-208). New York: Academic Press.

Lazarus, R.S. (1991). Progress on a cognitive-motivational-relational theory of emotion. *American Psychologist, 46,* 1019-1024.

Locke, E.A. (1995). Beyond determinism and materialism, or isn't it time we took consciousness seriously? *Journal of Behavior Therapy and Experimental Psychiatry, 26,* 265-273.

McClelland, D.C., & Kirshnitt, C. (1988). The effect of motivational arousal through films on salivary immunoglobulin A. *Psychology and Health, 2,* 31-52.

Michelson, L. (1986). Treatment consonance and response profiles in agoraphobia: The role of individual differences in cognitive, behavioural, and physiological treatments. *Behaviour Research & Therapy, 24,* 263-275.

Miller, J.G. (1978). *Living Systems.* New York: McGraw-Hill.

Mohl, P.C. (1987). Should psychotherapy be considered a biological treatment? *Psychosomatics, 28,* 320-326.

Natsoulas, T. (1978). Consciousness. *American Psychologist, 33,* 906-914.

O'Brien, J.T., & Arnes, D. (1994). Editorial: Why do the depressed elderly die? *International Journal of Geriatric Psychiatry, 9,* 689-693.

Öst, L.G., Jerremalm, A., & Johansson, J. (1981). Individual response patterns and the effects of different behavioural methods in the treatment of social phobia. *Behaviour Research & Therapy, 19,* 1-16.

Öst, L.G., Johansson, J., & Jerremalm, A. (1982). Individual response patterns and the effects of different behavioural methods in the treatment of claustrophobia. *Behaviour Research & Therapy, 22,* 445-460.

Pennebaker, J.W. (1993). Putting stress into words: Health, linguistic, and therapeutic implications. *Behaviour Research & Therapy, 31,* 539-548.

Pennebaker, J.W., & Beall, S. (1986). Confronting a traumatic event: Toward an understanding of inhibition and disease. *Journal of Abnormal Psychology, 95,* 274-281.

Pennebaker, J.W., Kiecolt-Glaser, J.K., & Glaser, R. (1988). Disclosure of traumas and immune function: Health implications for psychotherapy. *Journal of Consulting and Clinical Psychology, 36,* 239-245.

Pert, C.B. (1987). Neuropeptides: The emotions and bodymind. *Noetic Sciences Review, 2,* 13-18.

Petrie, K.J., Booth, R.J., Pennebaker, J.W., Davison, K.P., & Thomas, M.G. (1995). Disclosure of trauma and immune response to a Hepatitis B vaccination program. *Journal of Consulting and Clinical Psychology, 63,* 787-792.

Plutchik, R. (1994). *The Psychology and Biology of Emotion.* New York: Harper Collins.

Schleifer, S.J., Keller, S.E., Bartlett, J.A., Eckholdt, M.M., & Delaney, B.R. (1996). Immunity in young adults with major depressive disorder. *American Journal of Psychiatry, 153*, 477-482.

Schwarz, G.E. (1984). Psychobiology and health: A new synthesis. In B.L. Hammond, & C.E. Scheirer (Eds.), *Psychology and Health* (pp. 145-193). Washington, DC: American Psychological Association.

Schwarz, G.E., Davidson, R.J., & Goleman, D.J. (1978). Patterning of cognitive and somatic processes in the self-regulation of anxiety: Effects of meditation versus excercise. *Psychosomatic Medicine, 40,* 321-328.

Shevrin, H., & Dickmann, S. (1980). The psychological unconscious: A necessary assumption for all psychological theory? *American Psychologist, 35,* 421-434.

Sperry, R.W. (1969). The modified concept of consciousness. *Psychological Review, 76,* 532-536.

Surman, O.S., Williams, J., Sheehan, D.V., Strom, T.B., Jones, J.K., & Coleman, J. (1986). Immunological response to stress in agoraphobia and panic attacks. *Biological Psychiatry, 21,* 768-774.

Teasdale, J.D., Segal, Z., & Williams, J.M.G. (1995). How does cognitive therapy prevent depressive relapse and why should attentional control (mindfulness) training help? *Behaviour Research & Therapy, 33,* 25-39.

Vaillant, G.E. (1986). Empirical Studies of Ego Mechanisms of Defense. Washington, DC: *American Psychiatric Press.*

Van Rood, Y.L., Boogaards, M., Goulmy, E., & Van Houwelingen, H.C. (1993). The effects of stress and relaxation on the **in vitro** immune response in man: A meta-analytic study. *Journal of Behavioral Medicine, 16,* 163-181.

Van Rood, Y., & Goulmy, E. (1990). Stress, relaxation and changes in the immune system. In M.G.T. Kwee (Ed.), *PsychoTherapy, Meditation, and Health* (pp. 276-288). London: East-West.

Von Bertalanffy, L. (1968). *General System Theory.* New York: Brazillier.

Wiedenfeld, S.A., O'Leary, A., Bandura, A., Brown, S., Levine, S., & Raska, K. (1990). Impact of perceived self-efficacy in coping with stressors on components of the immune system. *Journal of Personality and Social Psychology, 59,* 1082-1094.

Zukav, G. (1979). *The Dancing Wu Li Masters.* New York: Morrow.

THE COMMON GROUND BETWEEN TWO GREAT WISDOM TRADITIONS: MAHAYANA BUDDHISM & CHRISTIANITY: WHAT CAN PSYCHOLOGY LEARN?

Mark Blows, M.A. (Hons),
Clinical Psychologist, Kenthurst, Australia

In the age of electronic media, internet and E-mail, effective communication between people of different philosophical traditions in still very slight, despite some progress. There is a better chance of this now than at other times in history. Previous beginnings of dialogue included the discussion at the court of Akbar The Great, The Sixteenth Century Mughal Emperor of India: the debates between Hindus and Buddhists at the University of Nalanda, India, eighth to twelfth centuries, and as reflected in the Islamic Sufi and Jewish Kabbala mystical movements, each with a long history but stimulated by the cultural contacts in Spain before the conquest of the Moors. Stephen Batchelor, The Awakening of the West, gives an account of the tragic misunderstandings and lost opportunities that occurred in the history of contacts between Christains and Buddhists in the Far East. Such misunderstandings and missed opportunities still occur but a notable recent exception is the very productive dialogue between the X1Vth Dalai Lama of Tibet, the Benedictine, Fr. Laurence Freeman and others at the 1944 John Main Seminar, Middlesex University, London. The history of exploration, leading into the historic dialogue at the John Main seminar, includes the work of Henry Le Saux, Bede Griffiths and the South Indian Benedictine monk and yoga master, Swami Amaldas, in respect of Hindu thought, and the American monk, Thomas Merton, in respect of Mahayana Buddhism.

Enclaves protect rigid adherence to particular traditions without understanding the similarities and the differences that exist between the various viewpoints. This unhealthy state of ignorance is a seed bed for indifference and conflict. We live at a time when it is relatively easy, at least in the 'developed' countries, to learn what our neighbour believes and practices.

I see the work of the Transnational Network for the Study of Physical, Psychological and Spiritual Wellbeing to be that of fostering effective communication between the wisdom traditions as well as that of using contemporary scientific skill to translate the values of those traditions into effective action in education and therapy. In this paper, I discuss two wisdom traditions, Mahayana Buddhism and Christianity and what psychology has done and can do with the teaching and concepts of these traditions.

The reasons for my choice are my own cultural background and the particular teaching that I have enjoyed.

In this dialogue it is important to understand that we are interdependent. The late Bede Griffiths wrote:

"We are realising today that no religion can stand alone" (River of Compassion, 1987, page 1).

I have suggested an amendment of this statement to read:

We are realising today that no religion can stand alone; so psychology cannot stand apart from the ethics of religion, nor religion ignore the practical wisdom of psychology (Proceedings of the Workshop: Towards the Whole Person, ed Mark Blows, 1993, cover sheet).
There is no possibility of examining all of the concepts of a wisdom tradition in one short paper. I have taken the key concepts of wisdom and compassion, together with one of the principal means for achieving these, meditation. Psychology enters the picture in two ways; experimental psychological studies and educative actions such as psychotherapy and counselling. There is also a pervading philosophical issue in the background of this area of study that should not be ignored and that is the Renaissance revolution that provided the conditions for humanistic science. The wisdom traditions rely to some degree on authority; psychology relies in theory at least on experimental demonstration, in experimental psychology or, at least, on the test of personal experience in its educative work. Any comparative study that includes psychology has to deal with this Gordian knot.

1) The Key Concept of Compassion

Compassion is not a theoretical construct in psychology. Love and compassion are hardly dealt with in the psychological literature, except in the notion of empathy and in the facilitation of wholeness in our clients in clinical work, in humanistic psychology.
Compassion is assumed by clinicians partly because people such as Carl Rogers were religious and partly because there is a vestige of religious thought, frequently Christian or Jewish, among practising psychologists. There is no necessary connection between compassion and psychology, as may be seen in some applications in the competitive world of commerce and industry and in some military applications. Compassion is the key concept of Mahayana Buddhism and Christianity as shown by the models provided by Gautama Buddha (Shakyamuni Buddha after enlightenment) and Jesus. The essential feature of compassion is a strong desire and commitment to bring suffering to an end.
Compassion is inherent in the four noble truths of Shakyamuni Buddha, the fact of suffering, the causes of suffering, cessation of suffering, and the means of cessation of suffering. The four noble truths were the basis for his very creative assistance to individuals that may be recognised today to include cognitive behavioural therapy, based on focussing of attention on pertinent aspects of personal behaviour and corrective self directed action (See Padmal de Silva, 1984, 1985, 1990). They were primarily the basis for

methods of transformation. Mahayana Buddhism emphasises the aspiration to become Buddha oneself, to be in touch with one's Buddha mind to help all sentient beings to attain Buddhahood a lofty and idealistic aim. Whereas Shakyamuni Buddha was happy for his immediate disciples to become Arhats, that is continuously mindful and liberated from habitual reflexive action, the Mahayana aim is to do both that and to aspire to assist all sentient beings to attain Buddhahood. As put well by Thich Nhat Hanh (1995), we are guided by the northern star, as it were, but we may not reach the star. Such an attitude greatly enriches the meaning of one's individual life and has great implications for all kinds of practical action such as conflict resolution, peace making, sharing of the world's resources, care for the habitat of animals, sustainable conservation and so on. It is not just pious ritual, although the Mahayana tradition is replete with rituals and imaginative mind training exercises.

There is a sticking point in this notion of compassion. According to Geshe Loden (1993), in his very comprehensive compendium on the graduated path, lam rim, of Tsong Khapa, the aim of compassion in Mahayana Buddhism is liberation of all sentient beings from cyclic existence. This appears to be a negative aim, perhaps consistent with the medieval Christian aim of deliverance from life in the body, an object of mortification, but hardly consistent with the emphasis in the Creational Theology of Matthew Fox nor, of course, the Renaissance attitude of joy in the beauty of life for its own sake. A possible way through this sticking point is provided by Sogyal Rinpoche (1992) who emphasises that the bardo state (experience after death) is the state that we have now. In other words, it is the internal attitude that matters, echoing the Christian idea that the kingdom of God is within and the Buddhist idea that the pure lands are a state of mind, now. Being alive in the present moment, totally mindful, grounded in that moment, whether it be a painful or pleasant one, fits all three traditions, I believe. (See Bousfield, 1996, for a practical guide in the field of pain management). We are frequently ruminating on the past or worrying about the future. Mindfulness is one of the keys to cessation of suffering. We may see Jesus's teaching about letting go of anxiety, caring not for future needs but trusting in providence, as pointing in the same direction.

Historical Background

In understanding the different traditions it is helpful to be aware of history, the context in which they arose. This is rarely encouraged by the teachers of particular traditions. In everyday colloquial language we acknowledge the importance of 'understanding where we are coming from'.

Buddhism has its origins in the Hindu thought and practice of ancient India. The Patanjali sutras or teaching, compiled under the name of a person called Patanjali, have a generic status in this history. It is be a moot point about which set of sutras came first, those of Buddha or Patanjali. There was a common heritage. In Patanjali's system, which is still very alive in India today, there is emphasis on ethics as the basis of training. This carried over into Buddhism. Included in both, for example, are ahimsa (non- violence), asteya (not stealing), aparigraha (living simply without hoarding) and bramacarya (highest conduct, including but not limited to responsible sexual conduct).

Buddhists will recognise these as essential precepts and it is obvious to persons of the Syriac traditions, Jews, Moslems and Christians that these precepts are part of the Mosaic law. These ethical rules became internalised as attitudes or orientations in the more sophisticated interpretations, thus Karambelkar (1985-1987) was able to give a more subtle interpretation to ahimsa for example, even to the point of being gentle to those who require our help, thus touching on compassion, and going beyond the original precept of not killing (which is still part of the notion). Starting with the Patanjali background, Shakyamuni Buddha was able to revolutionise yoga from its original emphasis on a dualistic separation of Purusha (supreme spirit within) from prakriti or material world, to realisation of compassion within a setting of interdependence.

Jesus reformulated Mosaic law to a more internalised, attitudinal form so that, for instance, covetous attitudes rather than overt acts such as sexual misconduct and stealing were emphasised. The opposite to the notion of "loving our neighbour as ourself" is what Buddhists call ego grasping.

Western psychology has a very different history. Psychologies of various kinds, are, of course, as old as man's reflection on himself and are found in many different cultures. The word 'psychology' is usually assumed to mean western psychology and frequently Anglo-American psychology. It has its origins in the dualism of Descartes.

For convenience, in order to avoid conflict with the dogmas of the Church, he conceived mind and matter as separate spheres. Mind stuff was allotted to the Church and matter stuff was allotted to science. This history has been reviewed very fully by Professor Paranjpe, a migrant to the west who was awake to the differences of viewpoint. I thoroughly recommend his book, Theoretical Psychology: The Meeting of East and West (1984) for a serious study of this issue as it has affected psychology. He re- evaluates the old issue of introspection, based on the mistaken idea ofTitchener that experience could be analysed into components like chemicals into atoms. Introspective data were never rejected in Indian psychology. The Western attitude has led to great expertise in experimental design and statistical analysis for quantitative measurement but ethics and compassion, without which applied psychology lacks adequate purpose, do not emerge from experimental designs. In my opinion, psychology is not sufficient within itself. It is appropriate to take account of its relationship with the wisdom traditions, accepting our interdependence.

2) The Key Concept of Wisdom

Wisdom has many meanings but two that I wish to concentrate on here are attachment, realisation of interdependence or the opposite side of that coin, emptiness.

I prefer to use the word non- attachment rather than detachment because the latter has connotations of schizoid non- involvement. Since the Shakyamuni Buddha revolution, non- attachment is no longer confined to the older notion of separation. Compassion introduces a new dimension of meaning that is not dualistic. This is a re-casting of the basic religious process of renunciation. A notion of relatedness transforms the purpose of renunciation, especially in Mahayana.

Non- attachment is a very complex notion. The psychologist, Derek Roger (1995a,

1995b, 1996a, 1996b, Roger & Jamieson, 1988, Roger & Najarian, 1989, Roger, D.B. & Nesshoever, 1987, Roger & Schapals, 1996, Roger et al, 1993, Roger et al, 1994) has captured part of it in a factorial dimension based on the idea of rumination. It goes beyond the absence of unproductive rumination, however. Attachment includes identification of action with desire. If a person is very 'cool' and seldom ruminates but is devoted to his own fame or position in one or other of our society's hierarchies, then that person would be in a condition of attachment. Jesus, in his teaching, as translated into various languages, never used the word non- attachment yet this is the very essence of much of his teaching. Take for example the story of the rich man who followed most of the precepts of right conduct but who could not deal with the challenge of on attachment (the parable of the camel proceeding through the eye of the needle) or the Sermon on theMount. In Buddhism desire is seen as one of the three poisons; hatred, which is derived from frustration of desire, and ignorance (being blinded by concepts such as those used in the service of attachment or aversion) being the other two. Frustration and lamentation are the suffering that follow from the loss of the objects of attachment. Like love and compassion, attachment colours conduct without being easily isolatable or abstracted from a context. So, although Derek Roger is doing very well to extract the dimension of attachment, detachment as he prefers to call it, from his mathematical-statistical method, there is a long way to go before there is complete correspondence. Like other contemporary attempts to reproduce yogic concepts in experimental psychology, it is, as Bede Griffiths would say, "good as far as it goes" but does not yet capture the full meaning. That, of course, need not worry the clinician very much because he or she does not rely on experimental models, only using them when and if they are available for the practical challenge at hand. For the clinical psychologist or educator who sees his work as part of a wisdom tradition, Derek Roger's work is, nevertheless, encouraging.

The linch pin of wisdom, in the Mahayana path, is realisation of interdependence or emptiness. It is regarded as 'strong meat' and should not be taught to those who are not ready to assimilate it and for whom it may have a destabilising effect.

There are various logical arguments used to support the key notion of emptiness. I have some difficulty with these, even though Geshe Loden (1993) claims that they produce absolute certainty. Intuitively, the notion is self evident. Logic, involving as it does the manipulation of words invites counter-arguments and it is not so difficult to produce them. Space does not allow for a critique of these arguments here. They are put well by Geshe Loden. I shall present one that he does not emphasise and then move onto an intuitive appreciation. The arguments are part of Madhyamika philosophy, presented often by the Dalai Lama. If we take an object such as a chair, for example, where, according to the argument, lies the inherent existence of that chair; in its legs, seat and so on? It is shown that the chair cannot be located in any of its parts. What this argument fails to concede, in some versions of it, is that the chair is a constellation. The idea of constellation is not denied, in Madhyamika philosophy. The chair, for instance, would be regarded as an arbitrary arrangement, a conventional device developed in certain cultures, dependent on the carpenter's actions and the shape of the human body in a certain restful posture. The concept "chair" is a conventional ascription to an object that arose from various causes and conditions. This is a more sensible approach than the Platonic one towards concepts. The Dalai Lama (Kiely, 1996, p. 104) sets out three ways of understanding interdependence, linear causality, mutual dependence and emergence depending on context and environment. What emerges is not absolute, nor has it inherent existence from its own side.

At least the argument is better than the Platonic one in which perfect concepts exist and are laid up in heaven. That makes no sense at all. A chair is a chair by conventional ascription and there is some sense in the idea that it has no inherent existence. The notion is better illustrated by biological events. A flower, for example, has no inherent existence. It is an outcome of certain short term events at the end of a stalk, that depends on a vast interaction of events from genetic encoding processes to photosynthesis, favourable conditions of warmth, water, air, the presence of various nutrients in the soil, the action of worms, possibly favourable fungi and so on. If I take myself as an example, the notion is also obvious. In four minutes without oxygen I would have irreversible brain damage. I depend on continual consumption of water, digestion of food, and so on. My thoughts emerge because of parental influences, various teachers, culture and accidents of experience. The essential me- ness is not my legs, my arms nor any parts, nor thoughts, neither is it my psychological identity. My identity is constantly in flux, even if there is a certain substratum of temperament that endures but even that is changing with age.

Professor Paranjpe would agree with this so far but might be tempted to say that my witnessing of the story of my life, that intangible Purusha is the only part that has inherent existence. Even that is in question. That atman (self) is an-atman (non- self) according to Shakyamuni Buddha; it may emerge as a temporary structure under certain conditions only. In short the idea of emptiness may be readily appreciated. The notion emptiness/interdependence is one of the very helpful ones in Mahayana Buddhism.

Thich Nhat Hanh (1995, page 184) writes:

"Non- self is also interdependence. Nothing can be by itself alone. It has to inter-be with all other things. This is non-self."

The only point I wish to add is that, in our climate of post quantum physics it is best to emphasise events rather than things. A flower is an event, even the chair is an event, i.e. a relatively slowly changing pattern or a slowly changing structure if taken as a thing. Christian contemplative writing on the noumenon suggests realisation of emptiness.

For example, the church father John Cassian who inspired John Main (1980, 1989) and Laurence Freeman (1986, 1989) in their development of Christian Meditation, espoused dropping of all images and the boundaries of self. In one sense boundaries of the self are dropped, with an attitude of apatheia (Freeman, 1986, p 48), desirelessness and non- possessiveness, simplicity, neither aware of egoism or sanctity. In another sense, boundaries are not absent, there is not a sinking into torpidity, laxity, to use the Tibetan Buddhist term, rather increased alertness, so the person is very much present, despite the dropping off of psychological clutter. Boundaries are dropped in the sense that simplicity permits inter-being, in the Christian context, resting in God or the ground of being. In the higher Buddhist yogas, a union of one's child luminosity with the mother Luminosity is spoken of or, as put by the Dalai Lama, being of "one taste" with the dharmakaya (Kiely 1996, P. 105- 106), which is the parallel term for round of being. It is suggested in the writing of the unknown author of the medieval English work The Cloud of Unknowing who rejected what were known later as the categories of Kant as applying to the noumenon. Jesus spoke of the inter- being with the father, a symbol of the sky god, from the Greek colonial culture of his time. He also spoke of interdependence in one of his familiar agricultural symbols that of 'the vine and its branches', the body of the church with himself as the trunk.

The vine touches on one of the most common symbols of interdependence with each other and the noumenon. The Tree of Life, found almost universally in religion, eg. medieval Christian and Mahayana Buddhist refuge trees, in Australian Aboriginal, American Indian, Jewish Kabbala and Moslem mysticism (See Johanna Blows, 1995, for the Australian Aboriginal context). Once discovered in Buddhism, interdependence, may be recognised in Christianity- as also in Judaism, with the phrase "I am", attributed to Yahweh, expressed to Moses. Modern man is not comfortable with the notion of interdependence, because of our over- valuation of individualism. Western psychology has not favoured the idea of dying to the self in order to experience greater life in inter-being. It has promoted individual competition and ambition. Japan and other eastern countries, as well as Africa, for that matter (Saito, 1994), still carry interdependence as part of their general philosophy. In Japan, there is great emphasis on fitting in with society, rather than asserting oneself independently. Psychologies tend to reinforce the values of the cultures from which they arise. Denial of interdependence leads to suffering. In Buddhism, it is emptiness of inherent existence that permits change and spiritual growth and enables compassion. For example, acting generously one realises that, in a sense, there is no giver, nothing being given and no person receiving. One can also be generous because, had conditions been different we could be in a similar position to our enemy. It is realisation of emptiness that allows us to appreciate Jesus' sermon on the mount. It is a principal cause of the cessation of suffering, producing peace within the person and in society.

Meditation

Meditation is a method or process for developing wisdom and compassion.

Psychologists have gone to town on it, having taken it out of context and reified it.

In the 1970's it was the neurophysiological correlates that were studied intensively. It would take us too far afield to cover the various theories that emerged at that time. Sufficient to say that the construct of a hypometabolic state proved to be simplistic. Neither is synchronised alpha rhythm a necessary correlate of meditation. Both of these conclusions are shown in the work done under the direction of Akishige (1977) at Komazawa University, Tokyo, Japan. As explained frequently by the Dalai Lama, meditation requires the right balance between an active and a passive or relaxed mental state.

Since that time there have been useful clinical studies in Australia on the effectiveness of meditation in reducing cognitive anxiety. Before we have a brief look at this research, it is necessary to return to the meaning of meditation in the wisdom traditions. It is hardly possible for one person to grasp all the various meanings of meditation in the wisdom traditions. The basic mindfulness exercises in Early Buddhism provide one of the main foundations; the Hindu Yoga Sutras of Patanjali provide another important foundation. The Patanjali Sutras are an eight-fold path that leads into various stages of samadhi. This process is called samatha in Early Buddhism and it is the same method that leads into calm abiding which is a preparation for realising emptiness in the graduated path, lam rim, of Tsong Khapa. It is when we are under threat, when someone is angry with us or we angry with them that we are likely to lose the perspective of inter- being, an- atman. The steadiness that arises from the experience of loss of distance between seer and the object helps to realise emptiness. Patanjali called this phase samadhi nirbiji, or seedless meditation. When carried into everyday life our view is sharpened, as in Zen[1] wich is part of the Mahayana tradition.

In Zen, meditation is called "za3en"[2]. The recommended posture is the same as in Patanjali's Sutras, the lotus or half lotus, but there is no object of meditation, meditation is "nirbiji". Patanjali's sutras assume the dualistic samkhya philosophy but the technique does not really depend on that.

Judging from the description of calm abiding given by Geshe Loden (1993) the similarity is quite clear- there is direct continuity between the Hindu and Buddhist traditions in the use of samadhi. Any object at all may be used but both in the Patanjali sutras and in Geshe Loden's version of lam rim, the graduated path, a deity is recommended. Buddhists usually use Shakyamuni Buddha or one or another Buddha, including Tara the feminine version, or a Bodhisattva. For a Christian, the Virgin Mary or Jesus would be a suitable object, realising, in both cases, Buddhist and Christian, that the object is only an image. The breath is also an acceptable object. It is far from being an easy technique to master. The setting or context should be noted. Contemplatives do not meditate from a cold start. There is a ceremony, fixing a suitable environment, perhaps prostrations, perhaps other prayer, perhaps reading, perhaps mindfulness of the quality of some actions during the day, recognition of a klesha, or reflection on an act of kindness or cause of gratitude, perhaps the stylised ceremony of Soto Zen- but there is always a context for meditation. The context facilitates meditation and is not separate from it.

There is the slightly different technique that is used in the earlier form of Mahayana Buddhism in Tibet, the Nyingmapa Tradition. Here, the breath or a mantra may be used as the object of concentration but the attention is lightly, though steadily focussed. Thoughts are allowed to rise and fade, as clouds pass in the sky, perhaps noted but not energised with thinking. The seer neither indulges nor suppresses the thoughts, images or any mental products that might arise. Gradually, space appears between the thoughts and movements of mind, vittri, as Patanjali called them, cease. Once again there is alertness, a state of being awake, not dullness of mind.

There is a more basic technique in Buddhism and that is analytical meditation. This is virtually the same technique as the Benedictine method, of Lectio Divina, reading with the word. It is not so much a critical analysis but digestion of the text, reflection on its meaning and application, followed by silence. The silence could be regarded by a neu-

---

[5] In zen, meditation is called *zazen*. The recommended posture is the same as in Patanjali's Sutras, the lotus or half lotus, but there is no object of meditation, meditation is *nirbiji*. For a description of Zen training see Nakamura (1992) and Onda (1992).

ropsychologist as a sensible technique for consolidation of the memory of what has been studied. But it is more than that, the idea is to savour the teaching, to dwell with it and value it, feeling the presence even of the teacher behind the words. This general style of meditation is called meditation by the author of the Cloud of Unknowing while the silent concentration or samadhi is called contemplation- the opposite of current usage of the terms. Many exercises, using imagination, such as equalising liking, indifference and aversion to persons (an early exercise in the graduated path to counteract attachment) are also called meditation in Buddhism. This extends into the various tantric exercises of vajrayana, where energies are realigned by frequent practice. All this said and done, there is no reason at all why any experience in ordinary practical life may not be regarded as meditation. The beginner student needs time to practise in a simplified, untrammelled setting but the advanced student may use everyday experience- in fact mindfulness and calm abiding in daily life are the aim of practice. Bad experiences in life are especially good for alerting one to mindfulness and calm abiding. It is never recommended that life experiences be used only. Formal sitting sessions are continued.

The Benedictine monks, John Main and Laurence Freeman, discovered similarity between the method of meditation used by Cassian who inspired St. Benedict, and that used by the Hindu, Swami Satyananda, who taught Fr. John Main some years previously in Malaya (Freeman 1989, McKenty, 1987). This gave them courage to develop their version of Christian meditation. In this a mantra is used, as in the Jesus prayer of the Christian Orthodox Church. The mantra is maintained throughout the sitting session, "ploughing through" the distractions. In the writings of St John of the Cross and Meister Eckhart, the soul is said to maintain its search for God in darkness, that is without concepts. This may not be the same experience as samadhi nirbiji (seedless meditation) in Patanjali's Sutra but there is one important common element of experience and that is being awake or present. There is never an absence of attentiveness.

In experimental psychology new work has been done in Australia by Jagdish Dua (1989, 1992, 1993) and Ali Sahebi (1996, 1996a, 1996b). As their names might suggest both are immigrants and carry in their person cross cultural influences. Prof. Dua has studied many articles about meditation in various religions, and in the style of factor analysis or reduction to the simplest principle, has concluded that its essence is silence, absence of thought. From this abstraction, he, and later, Ali Sahebi (1996) have conducted experiments which show convincingly, that this 'meditation' is effective in reducing cognitive anxiety. This approach fits nicely with that of Derek Roger (ibid.), at York University, England, which is that the essence of detachment, a way to cessation of suffering and distress, is the cessation of rumination or agitated cogitation. From one point of view, these three people have provided us with a brilliant demonstration of the relevance and effectiveness of psychological processes crystallised from the wisdom traditions. Yet none of them claim that these outcomes of research are a sufficient rendition of the wisdom techniques of meditation or of the notion of detachment. Jagdish Dua advocates the full set of preparatory educational steps for meditation, as set out in Patanjali's Sutras (1993) and Ali Sahebi has referred to the meditation technique used in his experiment as "an attention control technique"(Sahebi & Menzies, 1996a, 1996b), rather than meditation. Derek Roger also acknowledges the limitations of what he has been able to crystallise in the experimental framework of personality questionnaire construction. This is not to disparage these attempts for it is truly gratifying to make realistic connections between experimental science and the wisdom traditions. It is obvious, I think, that the forms of 'meditation', used by Jagdish Dua and Ali Sahebi will become useful tools in cognitive- behavioural therapy. I have placed their work together because Ali Sahebi has drawn on the work of Professor Dua but their approach is not quite the same. Ali Sahebi's instructions for meditation, in his study, are very similar to those of the Nyingmapa method that I referred to above. In clinical practice, as distinct from experimental studies, it is also possible to increase flexibility in the instruction so that it is quite possible, according to the readiness of the client to move between the scientifically arrived derivatives and the approach of the wisdom traditions. This is what Johanna Blows and I had in mind in developing the 'Clenched Hand/Open Hand' (1989) technique for relaxation leading into meditation, drawing from the earlier work of Ron Farmer and from yoga. In Christianity meditation is a form of prayer, as it is at, least at a subtle level, in the Indian traditions. It is not appropriate to pray with (as distinct from praying for) people for whom prayer has no meaning. Therefore it is good to have secular derivatives to teach these persons how to reduce suffering. I also commend the sophisticated approach of Herbert Benson, of the Harvard Medical School who still uses his construct the relaxation response but appreciates the greatly varied ways in which tranquillity is obtained (Friedmann, 1993).

Guru Yoga

To enter fully into this vital topic would take us too far afield, but I cannot end this discussion without at least some mention of it. It is one of the most important ways of entering into the paths of both Mahayana Buddhism and Christianity, even if some people criticise Christianity because the root guru, Jesus is remote to them. There is a major issue, which, on the face of it, would seem to vitiate the concept. It is an expectation of contemporary men and women, at least those of us that have a scholarly background, to critically inquire into all ideas that teachers may put to us. Authoritative transmission is alien to us. I do not think that persons of Asian culture quite understand this, just as we find the concept of interdependence/emptiness difficult to grasp.

There are solutions to this problem, all that I can do here is to quote Shakymuni Buddha:

"Monks and scholars
Should well analyse my words,
As gold is tested by melting, cutting and rubbing,
Then adopt them, but not for the sake of showing me respect (Loden, 1993, p.570)."

This is an attitude that is completely consistent with the spirit of scientific enquiry. The relationship between master and student need not be a copy of that in Tibet nor of that in Japan. Many westerners alienated from their own culture, especially in the big counter culture movements in America, Australia and Europe after the Vietnam War, have identified themselves with Buddhism, suppressing their own cultural heritage. This may lead to false gains, based sometimes on anger, as when, for example, as reported by Batchelor, the founder of the Western Buddhist Order, Sangharakshita, encouraged blasphemy to cut ties with the Christian tradition.

Analyses based on sympathetic understanding, not hostile reactions are needed, just as sympathetic understanding is required for any creative action with psychologists' or psychotherapists' clients. Thich Nhat Hanh (1995), who suffered greatly in the Vietnam War, has provided a brilliant account of the similarities[6] of the two Wisdom Traditions that have been discussed here, based on his experience as a participant observer in both of them. Within reason, I favour looking for the commonalities between disciplines and traditions. Caution is required for two reasons. In any one tradition, there are contrary sub- traditions. The view of an- atman that I have presented here, for instance, is not the same in all Buddhist traditions and many Christians would prefer a much more personal view of God than that of the ground of being, which I prefer, and which is more resonant with the idea of the Dharmakaya. The second reason is as expressed humorously, very frequently, by the Dalai Lama: "One should not put a yak's head on a sheep's body". Concepts may appear to be the same but that can be deceptive. Psychologists have been able to define what they mean by detachment meditation. As shown, there is only a partial relationship between these concepts, used by them, and those in the wisdom traditions.

So, in the less operationally defined usages in the wisdom traditions, it is important to be alert to differences of meaning. Linguistic knowledge is helpful in this context.

I hope I have given a reasonably clear account, at least a pointer for further work on the common ground between the two wisdom traditions and the point that psychology has reached in its interaction with them up to the present time. I think we can be confident about adding the extra line to Bede Griffiths' statement about standing together, interdependence.

Acknowledgments

Somehow, I am not sure how, my wife Johanna spots the right books, those ones that I

[6] Within reason, I favour looking for the commonalities between disciplines and traditions. Caution is required for two reasons. In any one tradition, there are contrary sub-traditions. The view of *an-atman* that I have presented here, for instance, is not the same in all Buddhist traditions and many Christians would prefer a much more personal view of God than that of the *ground of being*, which I prefer, and which is more resonant with the idea of the *Dharmakaya*. The second reason is as expressed humorously, very frequently, by the Dalai Lama "One should not put a yak's head on a sheep's body". Concepts may appear to be the same but that can be deceptive. Psychologists have been able to define what they mean by *detachment* and *meditation*. As shown, there is only a partial relationship between these concepts, used by them, and those in the wisdom traditons. So, in the less operationally defined usages in the wisdom traditions, it is important to be alert to differences of meaning. Linguistic knowledge is helpful in this context.

need at a certain time. I very much appreciate her interest, suggestions and that knack of alighting on the right book.
I look back with gratitude to my various teachers, commencing with my parents, several Anglican priests, Tibetan teachers and colleagues in the contemplative disciplines, psychology and other healing professions.

Bibliography

Akishige, Y. (ed) (1977). *Psychological Studies of Zen,* 1 & 11, Komazawa University, Tokyo.

Batchelor, Stephen (1994). *The Awakening of the West,* Harper Collins, London.

Blows, Johanna (1995). *Eagle and Crow: An Exploration of an Australian Aboriginal Myth.*, Garland Publishing, New York & London.

Blows, Mark (ed) (1993). *Towards the Whole Person: Integrating Eastern & Western Approaches to Body-Mind Skills,* Linking Publications, Kenthurst, Sydney.

Blows, Mark & Blows Johanna (1989). *Clenched Hand/Open Hand: a Modern Version of an Ancient Yogic Relaxation Technique and its Uses in Psychotherapy; with Detailed Instructions on How to Use it,* Linking Publications, Kenthurst, Sydney.

Bousfield, Lyn (1996). Meditation and chronic pain, *Relaxation & Meditation,* , 1, 915, Newsletter of the Australian Branch of the Transnational Network for the Study of Physical, Psychological & Spiritual Wellbeing, Linking Publications, Kenthurst, Sydney.

de Silva, Padmal (1984). Buddhism & behaviour modification, *Behaviour Research and Therapy,* 661- 678.

de Silva, Padmal (1985). Early Buddhism & behavioural strategies for the control of unwanted intrusive cognitions, *The Psychological Record,* 433- 437.

de Silva, Padmal (1990). Self management strategies in Early Buddhism: A behavioural perspective. In, *Space In Mind: East- West Psychology & Contemporary Buddhism,* John Crook & David Fontana (eds), Elewen Books, Shaftsbury.

Dua, J. K. (1989). Effectiveness of Meditation and Cognitive Restructuring in Reducing Distress. In P. Lovibond & P. Wilson (eds), *Clinical and Abnormal Psychology* Elsevier Science Publisher, North Holland.

Dua, Jagdish (1992). Meditation as a Technique of Cognitive Behaviour Therapy. In Mark Blows & Saroja Srinivasan (eds), *Perspectives on Relaxation & Meditation,* Spectrum Publications, Melbourne, Australia.

Dua, Jagdish (1993). Meditation Training: Training to do What and How to do it? In Mark Blows (ed), *Towards the Whole Person: Integrating Eastern & Western*
Approaches to Body- Mind Skills, Linking Publications, Kenthurst, Sydney.

Freeman, Laurence (1986). *Light Within: The Inner Path of Meditation,* Darton, Longman & Todd, London.

Freeman, Laurence (1989). *The Selfless Self,* Darton, Longman & Todd, London.

Friedman, Richard (1993). *The Relaxation Response.* Paper given at the International Symposium: Comparative and Psychological Study on Meditation, Makuhari, Japan.

Griffiths, Bede (1987). *The River of Compassion: A Christian Commentary on the Bhagavad Gita,* Amity House, N.Y.

Gyatso, Tenzin (14th Dalai Lama of Tibet) (1982). *Kindness, Clarity and Insight,* Snow Lion Publication, Ithaca, N.Y.

Karambelkar, P. V. (1985-1987) The Scrialised Text: Patanjali Yoga, In, *Yoga Mimamsa, Kaivalyadhama,* 24, 1, 137-176, 2, 177-216, 3, 217-156, 4, 275-296: 26, 1 & 2, 297-432, 3 & 4, 433-546.

Kiely, Robert (1996). *The Good Heart: His Holiness the Dalai Lama Explores the Heart of Christianity - and of Hymanity*, Wisdom Publications, Boston.

Loden, Geshe Acharya Thubten (1993). *The Path to Enlightenment in Tibetan Buddhism*, Tushita Publications, Yuroke, Melbourne, Australia.

McKenty, Neil (1986). *In The Stillness Dancing: The Journey of John Main*, Darton, Longman and Todd, London.

Main, John (1980). *Word into Silence*, Darton, Longman & Todd, London.

Main, John (1989). *The Way of Unknowing*, Darton, Longman & Todd, London.

Nakamura, Shoji (1992). Zen Practice and Meditation. In Mark Blows & Saroja Srinivasan (eds) *Perspectives on Relaxation and Meditation*, Spectrum Publications, Melbourne, Sydney.

Onda, Akira (1992). Zen, Satori (enlightenment) and Creativity. In Mark Blows & Saroja Srinivasan (eds), *Perspectives on Relaxation and Meditation*, Spectrum Publications, Melbourne, Australia.

Roger, Derek (1995a). Emotional control, coping strategies and adaptive behaviour. In, *Stress and Emotion*, 15, 255-264.

Roger, Derek (1995b). The mechanics of stress: A model for the relationship between stress, health and personality. *5th International Stress Management Association Conference, Noordwijkerhout, The Netherlands,* March 1995.

Roger, Derek (1996a). Detachment: research & practice, *Relaxtion & Meditation*, 7, 1, 6-8, Newsletter of the Australian Branch of the Transnational Network for the Study of Physical, Psychological & Spiritual Wellbeing.

Roger, Derek (1996b). The role of cognitive rumination, coping styles, and self esteem in moderating adaptational responses to stress. *Paper presented at the 8th European Conference on Personality, University of Ghent, Belgium,* July 8-12, 1996.

Roger, Derek, Glyn Jarvis & Bahman Najarian 91993). Detachment and coping: The construction and validation of a new scale for measuring coping stretegies. *Personality and Individual Differences, 15,* 6, 619-626.

Roger, Derek, Bahman Najarian & Glyn Jarvis (1994). The interactive effects of emotion control and coping strategies on adaptive behaviour. *Paper presented at the British Psychological Society Annual conference, Brighton,* March 24-27, 1994.

Roger, Derek & Jamieson, John (1988). Individual differences in delayed heart-rate recovery following stress: The role of extraversion, neuroticism and emotional control. *Personality and Individual Defferences*, 9, 4, 721-726.

Roger, Derek & Najarian, Bahman (1989). The contruction and validation of a new scale for measuring emotional control. *Personality and Individual Differences,* 10, 8, 845-853.

Roger, D. & Nesshoever W. (1987). The contruction and preliminary validation of a scale for measuring emotional control. *Personality and Individual Differences*, 8, 527-534.

Roger, Derek & Schapals, Thomas (1996). Repression-sensitisation and emotion control. *Current Psychology* 15, 1, 30-37.

Sahebi, Ali (1996). Research report: Effectiveness of meditation and progressive relaxation in reducing performance anxiety. *Relaxation & Meditation*, 7, 1, 6-8, Newsletter of the Australian Branch of the Transnational Network for the Study of Physical, Psychological & Spiritual Wellbeing.

Sahebi, Ali & Menzies, Ross G. (1996a). The effects of relaxation and attention control therapy on worry. *Paper read at the International Congress on Stress and Health,* 5-8th October, Manly, Sydney, Australia, 1996.

Sahebi, Ali & Menzies, Ross G. (1996b). The relationship between Attentional dysfunction and worry in test anxious students. *Paper read at the International Congress on Stress and Health*, 5-8 October, Manly, Sydney, Australia, 1996.

Saito, Akiko (1994). Current State of Studies and Applications of Eastern Body-Mind Practices in Europe. In *Current State of Eastern Medicine Around the World,* The Advances Research Centre for Human Sciences, Waseda University, Tokyo.

Sogyal, Rinpoche (1992). *The Tibetan Book of Living and Dying,* Random Century Group, Sydney.

Thich Nhat Hanh (1995). *Living Buddha, Living Christ,* Riverhead Books, G. P. putnam's Sons, N.Y.

The Cloud of Unknowing, anonymous author (1973). William Johnston (ed), Doubleday ,N.Y.

WHAT DOES MEDITATION CHANGE?: MEASUREMENT OF COGNITIVE STYLES

Dr. Yosuke Sakairi,
Associate Professor, Tokoha Gakuen University Sizuoka, Japan

There is a wide difference between religious meditation as a discipline for enlightenment and "convenient",i.e. pragmatic meditation, as a means for health promotion. In psychological studies, although convenient meditation is often used as an experimental method, religious meditation is used as a basis for theory.

It is necessary to close this gap between method and theory. However, it is extremely difficult to make the experimental procedure coincide with the original religious meditation. Instead, the experimental procedure should be thought of as "meditation." Based on the results of previous studies, it is useful to rethink our theories of meditation.

At this time, empirical studies of meditation were reviewed and the following two points will be discussed: "What is 'meditation'?" and "What are the effects of 'meditation'?" Then, I will introduce two developed tests which measure the change in cognitive style induced by "meditation." Finally, I shall give a report on the studies which used one of these tests.

1. "Meditation" as a subject of empirical research

Between the years 1972-1993, 1,008 research papers in the Psychological Abstract included the keywords "meditation", "yoga", and "zen buddhism." Out of the 1,008, except for theoretical discussions, reviews, and clinical reports, 364 were empirical research papers. There was a wide range of meditation techniques used in these studies (see Table 1). The most frequently used technique was TM (53%). Combining TM with a TM-like mantra meditation technique (10%) produces a total of 63%. Therefore, in this discussion, TM-type meditation will be defined as "meditation."

There are two components of "meditation." The first is concentrating while consciously keeping a passive attitude. The second is deciding on a detailed personal manner which must be strictly followed.

Table 1: Meditations used in empirical studies

Transcendental meditation	161*	53%
Yoga	47	16%
Mantra meditation technique	31	10%
Zen	26	9%
Mindfulness meditation	9	3%
Tai chi, Qigong	7	2%
Buddhist meditation	7	2%
Christian meditation	4	1%
others (prayer, rite, etc.	10	3%

* Number of research papers in which the technique was used.

In the first component, TM practitioners are required to meditate naturally, with no effort towards concentration or self-control (Denniston, 1986). Benson (1976) considered a "passive attitude" or "let it happen" approach the most important thing in meditation. More than with active concentration, passive concentration requires various attitudes or skills (for example: receptivity, flexibility, etc.). Thus, "meditation" can be considered as a task to obtain such attitudes or skills.

The second component is deciding on a detailed personal manner or style. In most practices, an optimal manner is chosen which suits the practitioner's character and purpose. But in "meditation", there is only one, pre-decided manner. The TM practitioner must strictly follow the rules of mantra repetition, meditation duration, practice schedule, commencing and ending procedures, etc.. This approach is deeply embedded in eastern culture. In Japanese "do" means style or manner: For example, ken-do (the way of the sword); sa-do (tea ceremony); and ka-do (flower arrangment). Practitioners strive for self-control while following a set behavioral manner. The purpose of practicing "do" is not to learn how to defend yourself with a sword, how to serve tea, nor how to arrange flowers, but is self-cultivation. In the process the practitioner struggles to apply a set behavioral manner. He is aware of his own behavioral or cognitive pattern, and in breaking away from the old pattern, will obtain a new pattern. For the purpose of separating from the old pattern, a set behavioral manner, that is unfamiliar to the practitioner and has ambiguous results, is adequate. In this case, the practice of meditation is especially appropriate. In TM, the participant often receives positive feedback regarding his meditation experience. Such intervention reinforces his positive cognitive attitude.

2. Consistently proved effects of meditation

In previous meditation studies, two main effects were researched: induced altered states of consciousness (ASC) effects and physiological relaxation effects.

In studies concerning induced ASC effects, only 22% used TM as a meditation technique. Instead, various techniques of yoga, vipassana, and a hyper-arousal technique with hyper-ventilation were used. Although these intense and ecstatic methods often induce a deep ASC and mystical experiences, convenient meditation such as TM rarely induces such experiences during meditation. An investigation into the peak experiences ofTM practitioners (Sakairi,1992) showed that only 27 out of over 2,000 subjects had peak experiences, which were judged by using a checklist. Essentially, peak experiences and enlightenment suddenly happen in everyday life, not during meditation. The same investigation showed that 74% (20 out of the 27 practitioners) had peak experiences outside of meditation. In the case of Zen, enlightenment also happens during daily life. Deep ASC experiences during practice are seen to be of no value and are called ma-kyo. Basically, convenience meditation, such as TM, is not a means to induce deep ASC.

In studies regarding physiological relaxation effects, over half (56%) used TM as a meditation technique. Due to Wallace's (1970) influential study on hypometabolic states during meditation, TM is thought of as a relaxation technique. However, later studies by Benson (1975), Fenwick (1977), and Becker (1981), etc. were unable to confirm the same reduction in metabolism that Wallace had found. Many studies, e.g. by Walrath (1975), Curtis (1976), and Delmonte (1984), etc., conclude that, although TM has a relaxation effect, the degree of effect is no greater than that of other techniques or simple rest. Also, walking during practice is the preferred TM technique for children under 9 years old. This "walking meditation" shows that lowered metabolic states are not essential for TM.

Outside of the meditation state, as Holmes(1987) reviewed, most studies have not confirmed changed physiological responsivity under stressful conditions. But most importantly, the same subjects who did not undergo any physiological changes, reported a significant decrease in anxiety levels (Goleman & Schwartz,1976; Kirsch & Henry,1979; Griffiths,et al.,1981; Pagano & Warrenburg,1983, etc.). The effects of meditation are more easily confirmed by psychological measures, such as questionnaires and rating scales, than by physiological measures.

Table 2 shows what questionnaires were used in the study of meditation. The most frequently used questionnaire was on anxiety. The other 2 main questionnaires concerned introversion-extroversion and locus of control. Most of the studies did not find significant changes in intro-extroversion (Ross,1977; Abrams & Siegel,1978) and locus of control (Zaichkowsky & Kamen, 1978; Zuroff & Schwarz,1978) after meditation practice. On the other hand, studies regarding reduction in anxiety levels constantly confirmed significant changes (Dillbeck,1977; Zuroff & Schwarz,1978; Throll,1981, etc.).

Table 2: Questionnaires used in studies of meditation

State-Trait Anxiety Inventory	29*
Eysenck Personality Inventory	14
Rotter's Locus of Control Scale	13
Schwartz's Anxiety Questionnaire	8
Shostrom's Personal Orientation Inventory	8
Tellegen's Absorption Scale	7
16 Personality Factor Questionnaire	6
Epstein-Fenz Manifest Anxiety Scale	5
Marlowe-Crowne Social Desirability Scale	5
Tennessee Self-Concept Scale	5

* The number of research papers in which the questionnaire was used.

According to the meta-analysis of Eppley (1989), the difference between the experimental group and the control group's anxiety score reduction rate was greater in TM (0.70 SD) than in progressive relaxation (0.38 SD) or other meditation techniques (0.28 SD). However, in studies using experimental techniques similar to TM, there was no difference between the experimental group and the control group (Smith,1976; Boswell & Murray,1979;Fling et al., 1981). The anxiety-reduction effect that was confirmed in studies using the original TM technique, without controls, is due to the entire TM instruction system, not just the TM technique itself.

In conclusion, the consistently proved effects of "meditation" is only with "anxiety scores as measured by questionnaires, which are reduced by the entire TM instruction system." Self-report type questionnaires do not measure personality itself, but only one's self-cognition of personality. Therefore, the answer to the question, "What does 'meditation' change?" is that self-appraisal of personality is related to anxiety, and as this self-appraisal changes so does one's anxiety level.

3. Development of cognitive style measures: Introducing 2 tests.

Based on the idea that questionnaires scores are affected by one's cognitive style, original measures of cognitive style were developed. In previous studies of the cognitive styles of meditators, field independence was measured mainly by the embedded figures test (Pelletier,1974;Gelderloos, et al.,1987). Also, flexibility was measured by using the Stroop Color Word Test (Van Nuys,1973) and the anagram task (Dillbeck,1982). Not only established tests, but also further, specially made tests that measure cognitive styles, susceptible to change by "meditation", are needed. What kind of transitions in mental attitude or cognitive style have occured? Table 3 shows three different transitional attitudes during Autogenic Training (AT) (Sakairi,1993). In the short term practice ofTM, the same attitude changes are supposed to occur (from 1. Negative -- Positive; 2. Persistent -- Flexible; 3. Directive -- Passive).

Now, I will introduce the Selective Recognition Test for measuring a negative-positive cognitive style, and the Figure Matching Card Test for measuring a persistent cognitive style or perfectionism.

Table 3: Attitude transition during use of AT

Obstructive Attitude to AT	Short Term Transition	Long Term Transition
1. Negative	-- Positive	-- Neutral
2. Persistent	-- Flexible	-- Free
3. Directive	-- Passive	-- Receptive

1. "Selective recognition test (SRT) to measure positive-negative style"

Clear results could not be obtained from previous studies in which selective recall of positive and negative words were used to measure the positive cognitive style of meditators (Gelderloos,et al.,1987). One reason for this is that there are great differences between the memory abilities of individuals. Thus, I have developed a test in which cognitive style and memory ability are separated.

Selective Recognition Test

This test's purpose is to measure selective attention, memory, and cognitive tendencies with respect to positive and negative words describing personality:For example, gentle, honest, kind...as positive words; arrogant, crafty, selfish...as negative words. In this test, 10 positive and 10 negative words reflecting personality traits were randomly placed on a sheet of paper (4 distractors were also inserted: 2 words above the group, 2 words below) and presented to the subject to look at for 20 seconds. Then the subject was made to sit for one minute with eyes closed while mentally counting backwards. A check-list of 24 words was given to the subject, who checked just 10 words that he or she could confidently recognize. The ratio of positive words to negative words was measured.

This test is appropriate for measuring individual differences in cognitive styles, through the following three interpretations:

1. In this test, all words are presented at once and the subjects are free to look at any words they choose. Thus, the results of this test are not only affected by the selectivity in the memory process, but also by the attention process.
2. The subjects are required to recognize words from a checklist, with the possibility of words being chosen not by memory. Thus, the results are also affected by selectivity in the cognitive process.
3. All subjects are required to recognize just 10 words. Therefore, deviation in the data, caused by differences in ability, becomes minimal.

2. "Figure matching card-test (FMCT) to measure perfectionism"

The matching figures test was developed by Kagan, et al.(1964) in order to measure reflection-impulsivity cognitive style of children. There are two problems: a) ability and cognitive styles are not distinguished, and b) it is not adequate for adults. Therefore, a test was made which separates ability and cognitive style and is available for adults.

[Figure Matching Card Test]
The test measures the number of times and duration which the subject confirms the sameness of two figures (see Figure 1).

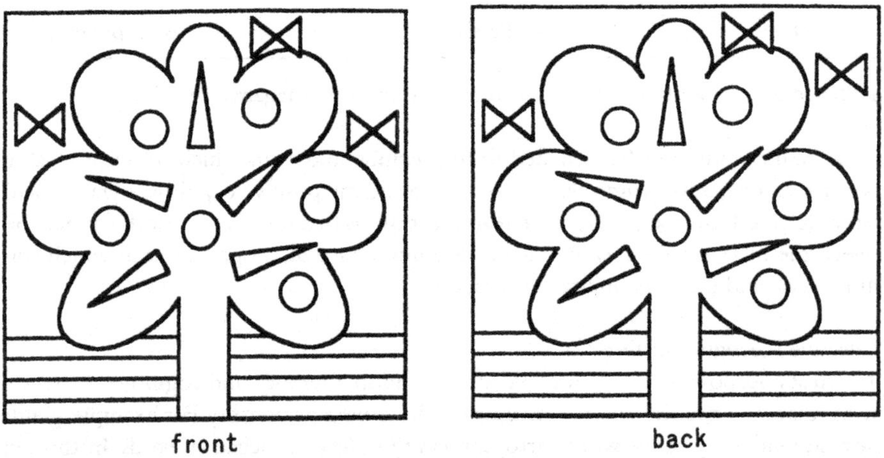

Fig. 1 Sample of figures used in FMCT.

For this test, 15 cards which had the same figure on the front side were used. From these cards, 8 cards had the same figure on the back. On the other 7 cards, one-part of the figure on the back side was different. The subject was required to determine if the front and back sides were the same or different with no errors. The length of time the subject took and the number of checks required for determination, was measured. Then, the score for perfectionism was obtained by subtracting the totals of the 7 different cards from the 8 identical cards.

When the subject is unable to detect any difference in figures that are identical, it is the subject's attitude, not ability, that influences whether or not he decides there is no difference, or continues to check, for the possibility that he has not found the difference yet. In this test, the results with the different cards are considered an ability related to detection. Therefore, this test is able to distinguish between perfectionism and detection ability.

4. Studies of selective-recognition style of meditators.

The cognitive style and anxiety levels of TM practitioners were investigated by using the Selective Recognition Test(SRT), the Form X-II of the State Trait Anxiety Inventory(STAI), and the Cattell Anxiety Scale(CAS).

Study 1: Selective recognition tendencies and trait-anxiety levels of long-term TM practitioners (Sakairi,1996).
Method: 83 meditators (49 males and 34 females) who practiced TM for an average of 2 years and 9 months and 102 non-meditators (72 males and 30 females) on a waiting list were tested using the SRT, STAI, and CAS.

Results: Meditators recognized more positive words on the SRT than non-meditators ($t=2.76$, $df=183$, $P<.01$) and showed lowered anxiety levels measured by STAI ($t=4.59$, $df=142$, $P<.001$) and CAS ($t=2.27$, $df=142$, $P<.05$); (see Table 4).

Table 4: Selective recognition and anxiety levels of TM practitioners

	SRT	STAI	CAS
TM Group	5.69	38.3	27.0
(SD)	(1.54)	(8.8)	(13.3)
Non-TM Group	5.06	43.4	33.0
(SD)	(1.53)	(10.2)	(13.2)
t-test	P<.01	P<.001	P<.01

Out of the 83 meditators, two groups were selected: The first group (positive) in which 23 people recognized 70% or more positive words, and the other group (negative) in which 17 people recognized 40% or less. The anxiety levels of the positive group were lower than that of the negative group in both the STAI ($t=2.67$, $df=38$, $P<.05$) and CAS ($t=2.27$, $df=38$, $P<.05$);(seeTable 5

Table 5: Anxiety levels of positive and negative group

	STAI	CAS
Positive Group	35.3	24.3
(SD)	(8.2)	(13.3)
Negative Group	42.5	35.3
(SD)	(8.2)	(16.3)
t-test	P<.05	P<.05

Study 2: Change in selective recognition tendencies and trait-anxiety levels before and after TM.

Method: 42 subjects (28 males and 14 females) were tested before and after 14 weeks of TM practice by using SRT, STAI, and CAS.

Results: The ratio of positive words recognized in the SRT increased after TM practice ($t=2.32$, $df=41$, $P<.05$). The anxiety levels decreased in both the CAS ($t=4.38$, $df=41$, $P<.001$) and the STAI ($t=4.59$, $df=41$, $P<.001$); (see Table 6). The increase in recognized positive words showed a significant correlation with the reduction of anxiety scores in both CAS ($r=-0.31$, $t=2.06$, $P<.05$) and STAI ($r=-0.35$, $t=2.36$, $P<.05$).

Table 6: Selective recognition and anxiety levels before and after TM

	SRT	STAI	CAS
Pre Test	5.14	43.7	33.2
(SD)	(1.50)	(8.5)	(13.3)
Post Test	5.79	38.3	23.5
(SD)	(1.77)	(8.4)	(12.8)
t-test	P<.05	P<.001	P<.001

Conclusions

1. What does "meditation" change? Self-cognition or self-evaluation of one's personality as related to anxiety.
2. Based on the idea that cognitive styles or mental attitudes are modified through meditation practice, two tests were developed in order to measure positive-negative cognitive styles and perfectionism.
3. The study using the selective-recognition test found that there was an increase in positive cognitive style after TM. This increase was also correlated with a reduction in anxiety scores.

References

Abrams, A.I., & Siegel, L.M. (1978). The Transcendental Meditation program and rehabilitation at Folsom State Prison: A cross-validation study. *Criminal Justice and Behavior*, 5, 3-20.

Becker, D.E., & Shapiro, D. (1981). Physiological responses to clicks during zen, yoga, and TM meditation. *Psychophysiology*, 18, 694-699.

Benson, H. (1976). *The relaxation Response*. New York: Avon Books.

Benson, H., Steinart, R.F., Greenwood, M.M., Klemchuk, H.M., & Peterson, N.H. (1975).

Continuous measurement of O2 consumption and CO2 elimination during a wakeful hypometabolic state. *Journal of Human Stress*, 1, 37-44.

Boswell,P.C.,& Murray,E.J. (1979). Effects of meditation on psychological and physiological measures of anxiety. *Journal of Consulting and Clinical Psychology*, 47, 606-607.

Curtis,W.D.,& Wessberg,H.W. (1976). A comparison of heart rate, respiration, and galvanic skin response among meditators, relaxers, and controls. *Journal of Altered States of Conciousness*, 2, 319-324.

Delmonte,M.M. (1984). Physiological concomitants of meditation practice. *International Journal of Psychosomatics*, 31(4), 23-36.

Denniston,D. (1986). *The TM Book*. Iowa: Fairfield Press.

Dillbeck,M.C. (1977). The effect of the transcendental meditation technique on anxiety level. *Journal of Clinical Psychology*, 33, 1076-1078.

Dillbeck,M.C. (1982). Meditation and flexibility of visual perception and verbal problem solving. *Memory and Cognition*, 10, 207-215.

Eppley,K.R.,Abrams,A.I.,& Shear,J. (1989). Differential effects of relaxation techniques on trait anxiety: A meta-analysis. *Journal of Clinical Psychology*, 45, 957-974.

Fenwick,P.,Donaldson,S.,Gillies,L.,Bushman,J.,Fenton,G.,Perry,I.,Tilsley,C., & Serafinowicz,H. (1977). Metabolic and EEG change during transcendental meditation. *Biological Psychology*, 5, 101-118.

Fling,S.,Thomas,A.,& Gallaher,M. (1981). Participant characteristics and the effects of two types of meditation vs. quiet sitting. *Journal of Clinical Psychology*, 37, 784-790.

Gelderloos,P.,Goddard,P.H.,Ahlstrom,H.,& Jacoby R. (1987). Cognitive orientation toward positive values in advanced participants of the TM and TM-Sidhi program. *Perceptual and Motor Skills*, 64, 1003-1012.

Gelderloos,P.,Lockie,R.J.,& Chuttoorgoon,S. (1987). Field independence of students at Maharishi School of the Age of Enlightenment and a Montessori school. *Perceptual and Motor Skills*, 65, 613-614.

Goleman,D.,& Schwartz,G.E. (1976). Meditation as an intervention in stress reactivity. *Journal of Consulting and Clinical Psychology*, 44, 456-466.

Griffiths,T.J.,Steel,D.H.,Vaccaro,P.,& Karpman,M.B. (1981). The effects of relaxation techniques on anxiety and underwater performance. *International Journal of Sport Psychology*, 12, 176-182.

Holmes,D.S. (1987). The influence of meditation versus rest on physiological arousal: A second examination. In N.A.West (Ed.), *The Psychology of Meditation* (pp.81-103). Oxford: Clarendon Press.

Kagan,J., Rosman,D.L.,Day,D.,Albert,J.,& Phillips,W. (1964). Information processing in the child: Significance of analytic and reflective attitudes. *Psychological Monographs*, 78, 1-37.

Kirsch,I.,& Henry,D. (1979). Self-desensitization and meditation in the reduction of public speaking anxiety. *Journal of Consulting and Clinical Psychology*, 47, 536-541.

Pagano,R.R.,& Warrenburg,S. (1983). Meditation: in search of a unique effect. In R.J.Davidson, G.E.Schwartz,& D.Shapiro (Ed.), *Consciousness and Self Regulation* (pp. 153-205). New York: Plenum Press.

Pelletier,K. (1974). Influence of transcendental meditation upon autokinetic perception. *Perceptual and Motor Skills*, 39, 1031-1034.

Ross,J. (1977). The effects of the transcendental meditation program on anxiety, neuroticism, and psychoticism. In D.W.Orme-Johnson & J.T. Farrow (Ed.), *Scientific Research on the Transcendental Meditation Program: Collected Papers. Vol.1* (pp.594-596). Switzerland: Maharishi European Research University Press.

Sakairi,Y. (1992). Peak experience: Its features and mental health of peak experienced meditators. *Japanese Journal of Hypnosis*, 36, 95-103.

Sakairi,Y. (1993). The effects of meditative methods as a practice for acquiring new response patterns. 1993 *International Congress of Health Psychology*: Proceedings, 209-212.

Sakairi,Y. (1996). Anxiety levels and selective recognition of meditators. *Journal of Human Sciences*, 8(2), 64-70.

Smith,J.C. (1976). Psychotherapeutic effects of transcendental meditation with controls for expectation of relief and daily sitting. *Journal of Consulting and Clinical Psychology*, 44, 630-637.

Throll,D.A. (1981). Transcendental meditation and progressive relaxation: Their psychological effects. *Journal of Clinical Psychology*, 37, 776-781.

Van Nuys,D. (1973). Meditation, attention, and hypnotic susceptibility: A correlational study. *International Journal of Clinical and Experimental Hypnosis*, 21(2), 59-69.

Wallace,R.K. (1970). Physiological effects of transcendental meditation. *Science*, 167, 1751-1754.

Walrath,L.C.,& Hamilton,D.W. (1975). Autonomic correlates of meditation and hypnosis. *American Journal of Clinical Hypnosis*, 17, 190-197.

Zaichkovsky,L.D.,& Kamen,R. (1978). Biofeedback and meditation: Effects on muscle tension and locus of control. *Perceptual and Motor Skills*, 46, 955-958.

Zuroff,D.C.,& Schwarz,J.C. (1978). Effects of transcendental meditation and muscle relaxation on trait anxiety, maladjustment, locus of control and drug use. *Journal of Consulting and Clinical Psychology*, 46, 264-271.

PROCESS OF SELF-ACTUALIZATION THROUGH PRACTICING THE JAPANESE MARTIAL ART AIKIDO

Dr. Yoshitaka Konno,
Professor of Psychology, Faculty of Human Science, Bunkyo University, Japan

PURPOSE

In recent years, the importance of the holistic approach, in which a human being should be apprehended as being a body-mind integrated entity, has been emphasized in the field of psychosomatic medicine, clinical psychology, health psychology, and special education. One of the basic concepts of the holistic approach is to establish self-actualization based on direct experience or awareness of one's own inner state.

For this purpose a variety of body or body-mind exercise programmes has been developed, such as "Somatics" (Hanna,1970) and "Movement Arts" (Kleinman, 1986). These programmes include the Alexander Technique, Feldenkrais Method, Zen meditation, Yoga, Qi-gong, Tai-chi and other types of eastern martial arts based body-work. These programmes have insisted on the role of body awareness or rather body-mind awareness for integrating body-mind into a harmonious state, establishing a highly organized and well-functioning self-image, and eventually realizing self-actualization.

Aikido is one of the Japanese Martial Arts. It is a system of pure self-defense derived from the traditional weaponless fighting techniques of Jujuts in its use of immobilizing holds and twisting throws, whereby an attacker's own momentum and strength are used against him. Morihei Ueshiba (1883-1969) is credited with the modern systematization of Aikido. After schooling in the various martial arts, Ueshiba drew upon the teachings of Sokaku Takeda (1860-1943), who taught the Daito Aikido system of Jujuts or Judo. Later he created the basic skills of Aikido self-defense as distinct from Jujuts. Since the 1960s Aikido has spread rapidly in many countries of the world.

Aikido practice usually takes an established form, or "kata", in which one partner takes the offensive role dealing blows or holds and the other deflects these using Aikido moves. Basically, relaxing muscular tension, concentrating on Tanden-breathing (Tanden is considered to be located in the lower abdominal region, as shown in Figure 1), maintaining "Shizentai" (natural posture) and repeating "kata" are the most essential parts for Aikido practice. This study is aimed at examining the effects of Aikido practice on the enhancement of self-control over inner activities, positive changes in self-image, and self-actualization.

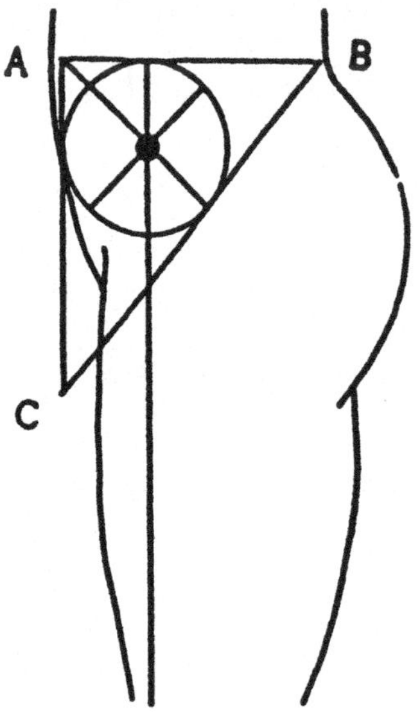

Figure 1. Location of Tanden in standing posture.

Method

1. Subjects

Forty-nine people (34 males and 15 females) who were continuously engaging in Aikido practice participated in this study. They were recruited from undergraduate students belonging to college Aikido club teams and people belonging to privately established groups for Aikido practice. The mean age of the subjects was 26 years and 7 months (ranging from 19.2 years and to 51.4 years). The average career of Aikido practice was 5 years and 8 months (ranging from 9 months to 30.2 years).

2. Questionnaire

To examine the effects of Aikido practice on the modification of self-image a 29-item questionnaire was used. These items were derived from the study of Howes (1987) and Konno (1989, 1990), and from the introspective reports collected from Aikido masters. These items comprised seven categories; Category 1: "attitude toward practice", Category 2: "awareness of body condition", Category 3: "progress of Waza (skill)", Category 4: "awareness of changes in personality and behaviour", Category 5: "attitude toward health management", Category 6: "self-acceptance", and Category 7: "acceptance of others".

Each item was evaluated using a five-point-rating scale comparing one's self-image from the beginning of the Aikido practice (beginning score) to the present time (current score).

Results

1. Factor analysis of questionnaire

The difference score ([current score]-[beginning score]) was calculated for each item, and then a factor analysis using the principal method was carried out. After Varimax-rotation the following factors were obtained (see Table 1). Factor 1: "fullness of mind-skill-body (shin-gi-tai)", Factor 2: "self-acceptance", and Factor 3: "acceptance of others". Factor 1 consisted of Categories 1 to 5. Factor 2 and Factor 3 corresponded to Categories 6 and 7, respectively.

2. Multiple regression analysis

Multiple Regression Analysis was carried out using mean difference scores in each category. As shown in Figure 2, significant relations were found between Category 1: "attitude toward practice" and Category 2: "awareness of body condition", as well as between Category 1 and Category 3: "progress of Waza (skill)". There was also a significant

Figure 2. Schematic representation of result of Multiple Regression Analysis.

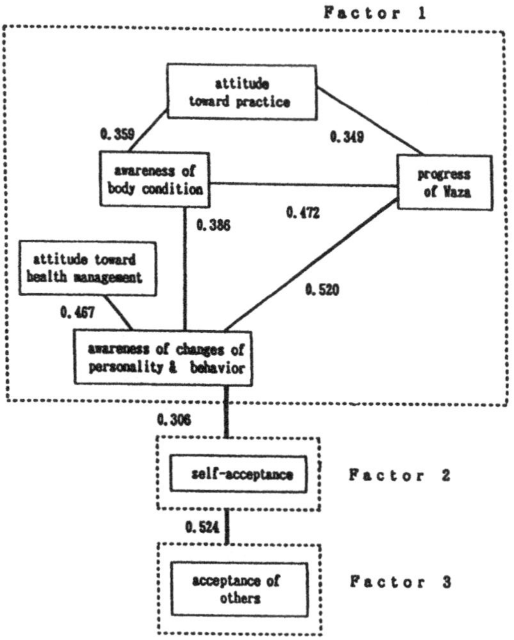

relation between Category 2 and Category 3. Both Category 2 and 3 related to Category 4: "awareness of changes of personality and behaviour", and in turn Category 4 significantly related to Category 6: "self-acceptance". Furthermore, Category 6 was significantly related to Category 7: "acceptance of others".

3. Comparisons of scores based on the career

According to the career of Aikido practice, subjects were assigned to three groups; Beginner group (N=20, from 9 months to 2 years of practice), Middle group (N=13, from 2.1 years to 5 years of practice), and Experienced group (N=16, from 5.1 years to 30.2 years of career). The mean age was 22 years for the Beginner group, 25 years for the Middle group, and 35 years for the Experienced group, respectively.

Figure 3 shows comparisons of difference scores among the three groups. As a result of One-Way Analysis of Variance, a significant difference was found for each category. Then, t-tests revealed significant differences between the Middle group and the Experienced group for Category 1, Category 2, Category 3, Category 5, and Category 7.

Figure 4 depicts comparisons of difference scores for each item among the three groups. Results of a One-way Analysis of Variance revealed significant differences for 23 of the 29 items. Results of t-tests yielded significant differences for 8 items between the Beginner group and the Middle group, for 26 items between the Beginner group and the Experienced group, and for 11 items between the Middle group and the Experienced group. These results indicated that the Experienced group excelled compared to the other groups in the following items: "relaxed attitude toward practice", "concentration on practice", "stability in blood pressure", "becoming cheerful and gentle", "behaving after careful consideration", "physical exercise to prevent disease", "doing cool-

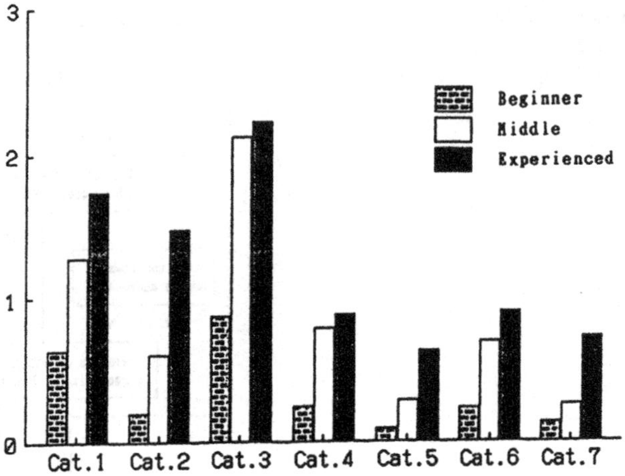

Figure 3. Comparison of mean differencen scores among three groups for each Category.

down exercise", "learning from mistakes", "esatblishment of emotional control", "providing help to person in need", and "recognizing another's good point".

Discussion

In this study, the author examined the effects of Aikido practice on the modification of self-image using a 29-item questionnaire. This questionnaire comprised 7 categories;Category 1:"attitude toward practice", Category 2:"awareness of body condition", Category 3:"progress of Waza(skill)", Category 4:"awareness of changes of personality and behaviour", Category 5: "attitude toward health management", Category 6:"self-acceptance", and Category 7:"acceptance of others".

Subjects were assigned to either a Beginner group, Middle group, or Experienced group according to their career in Aikido practice. Results indicated that a remarkable modification of self-image could be brought about as a function of one's career in Aikido practice. That is, the longer they experience Aikido practice, the better the changes in self-image that occur. However, in this study, a positive correlation was found between the length of Aikikdo practice and chronological age. Therefore, it was questionable whether the modification of self-image could solely be attributed to the length of practice. Since people might usually come to be more fully aware of themselves as they get older, the modification in self-image could be considered as a function of their life experiences. Neverthelss, the closer inspection of introspective reports concerning the changes in life-style provided clear evidence of the effects of Aikido practice on the modification of self-image.
Furthermore, Multiple Regression Analysis revealed that "fullness of mind-skill-body" (Factor 1) brought about "self-acceptance" (Factor 2), and in turn "self-acceptance" contributed to "acceptance of others" (Factor 3).
The process of modification of self-image or self-actualization found in this study was

Figure 4. Comparison of mean difference scores among three groups for each item.

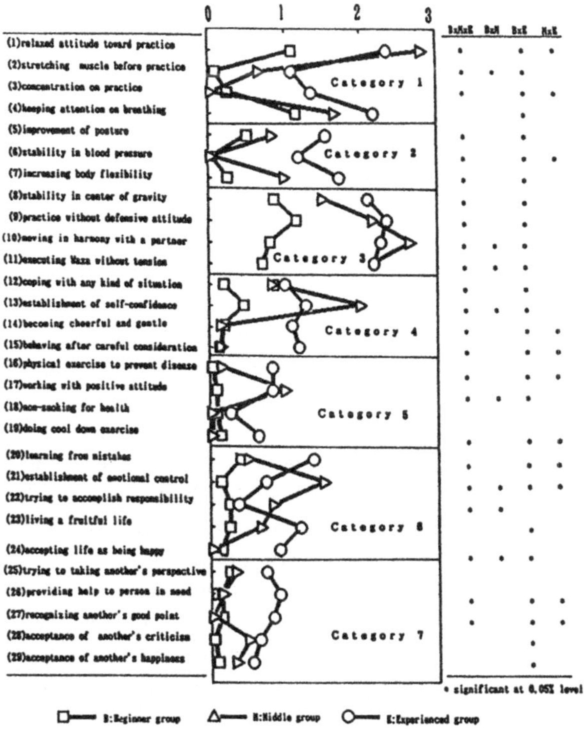

consisitent with the results of studies (Konno, 1989; 1990), in which the effects of Dohsa-method ("Psychological Rehabilitation" method) on the improvement of self-image or self-consciousness were examined. These studies have suggested that the experience of concentrating one's attention on good bodily sensations, abdominal breathing (especially for Tanden-breathing), postural states, and emotional states might play very important roles in becoming aware of one's own personality and behaviour, and in accepting both oneself and others.

As mentioned above, Aikido practice usually takes an established form or "kata", in which one partner takes an offensive role, e.g. dealing blows or special holds, and the other deflects these using Aikido moves. The success of these movements depends largely on the level of mutual understanding. Therefore, Aikido practice, performed in such a highly organized communicative situation, might help in learning to accept both oneself and others, and to take another's perspective.

References

Hanna, T. (1970): *Bodies in Revolt: A Primaer of Somatic Thinking.* New York: Holt, Rinhalt and Winston.

Howes, M.M. (1987): *Effects of physical fitness training on locus of control and the sense of wellness.* University Microfilm International.

Kleinman, S. (1986): *Somatics in higher education: The movement arts. Somatics*, Spring/Summer, 26-27.

Konno,Y.(1989): *On the Features in the Modification of Self-image through Muscular Relaxation(1). Annual Report of the Faculty of Education*, Bunkyo University, 23, 79-87.
Konno,Y.(1990): *On the Features in the Modification of Self-image through Muscular Relaxation(2). Annual Report of the Faculty of Education*, Bunkyo University, 24, 75-81.

Table 1. Questionnaire

Factor 1	Category 1: "attitude toward practice"
	(1) I approach practice in a relaxed manner and attitude.
	(2) I stretch before starting practice.
	(3) I concentrate my attention on body movement during practice.
	(4) I concentrate my attention on breathing during practice.
	Category 2: "awareness of body condition"
	(5) I feel my posture has improved.
	(6) I feel my blood pressure has come to be stable.
	(7) I feel my body flexibility has increased.
	Category 3: "progress of Waza (skill)"
	(8) I practice without defensive attitude or tension.
	(9) I execute body movement in accordance with that of my partner.
	(10) I keep my mind relaxed while executing Waza.
	Category 4: "awareness of changes in personality and behaviour"
	(11) I feel I can cope with any kind of situation.
	(12) I feel I have gained confidence through practice.
	(13) I feel my character has come to be cheerful and gentle.
	(14) I behave after considering the matter carefully.
	Category 5: "attitude toward health management"
	(15) I participate in practice to prevent disease.
	(16) I try to work with a positive attitude.
	(17) I avoid the use of tobacco for health purposes.
	(18) I cool down after vigorous exercise.
Factor 2	Category 6: "self-acceptance"
	(19) When I make mistakes I learn from them.
	(20) I can control emotion and anxiety.
	(21) I accept responsibility for my action.
	(22) I accept my life as being fruitful.
	(23) I can accept my happiness.
Factor 3	Category 7: "acceptance of others"
	(24) I make an effort to take another's perspective.
	(25) I provide reasonable help to a person in need.
	(26) I can accept another's good points.
	(27) I can express myself without defensive attitude.
	(28) I accept constructive criticism without reacting defensively.
	(29) I can accept another's happiness.

HOW TO USE TAOÏST MEDITATION TO ACCELERATE THE HEALING PROCESS

Nicole Tremblay, Ph. D., Ac.
Clinical Psychologist, Québec, Canada. Translated from the French by de I. de Boecklin and Marie Gèrin-Lajoie

1- Taoïst meditation: explanations and objectives

Taoïst meditation, " sitting in peace " (Ching Tsuo), is the basis of the Chinese and Asian knowledge of acupuncture and of the method of " mastering energy ", Qi Cong. It is used by the Taoïst masters firstly to perfect health and secondly to reach illumination. Taoïst meditation seeks the Wu Wei, the void, by observing nature and cooperating with it. To preserve his health, a man absorbs and keeps the sky's energy (Yang) and the earth's energy (Yin); he puts himself in harmony with the universe and pays attention to sensations in his body as a living and vibrating instrument. Wu Wei is also quietness, a state of inaction which is the source of all action. Tchouang Tseu stated: " Through inaction the sky clears up, the earth remains stable. Through the combination of sky, earth and inaction, all things operate... multiply and grow from inaction ".

Quietness is the result of meditation. Keeping the mind silent, not by stopping the constant flood of thoughts, but by keeping some distance from one's thoughts, by leaving intervals between thoughts, by acquiring a larger vision which includes respiratory sensation, body feelings, energy flow and physiological sensations, i. e. having feeling of all the senses at the same time. Quietness is the result of concentrating without effort on sensations instead of controlling thinking. In the Grand Teaching of the Tao it is said: " When one knows how to stop the thoughts, it is named concentration. Then one reaches quietness; and through quietness one acquires peace; and through peace, one reaches wisdom ".

Taoïst meditation is observing " what is ", outside and inside. Only " what is " remains, leaving behind duality, conflict, tòrmenting thoughts, judging and comparing. It is a global and holistic observation of life as a whole, as complete and indivisible; it is the observation of the motion of life, changing according to nature's laws, where man and universe vibrate together in unified energies. Master Mantak Chia says: " The Taoïst conception follows the models set by nature. We do not try to push our students to follow one method rather than another. Instead, we offer them a few different methods depending on their nature, capabilities and needs. The ultimate goal is to know oneself as we are, and to claim all our individual specificity at all levels, as our energy body, our energetic network is part of ourselves. All these Taoïst exercises help us discover and feel the Chi as a part of the human continuum: the energy of one's body, of the other bodies, of nature all around us ".

In " The Flame of Attention " Krishnamurti speaks also of meditation as observation with all the senses; through observing thought's motion, ego, consciousness, desire, time, violence, fear, image, conflict, faith, through observing all that makes us conditioned human beings, one reaches direct perception, timeless observation, and reaches, beyond those conditionings, true intelligence, light, compassion, and love. " Intelligence is the quality of sensitivity which perceives and acts with immediacy" (Krisnamurti, 1987).

Taoïst thinking influenced western thought through Carl Gustav Jung and his "Commentary of the Golden Flower Secret", through the bio-energetics of Wilheim Reich and Alexander Lowen, and through the transpersonnal psychology of Stanislav Grof. Many other modern methods such as sophrology, lucid dreaming, the Feldenkreis method, the Vittoz approach, and neurolinguistic programming seem to be inspired from oriental medicine and meditation.

Objectives of meditation

To reach an intelligence freed from contradictions, polemics, and argumentation coming from the ego, it is necessary to develop a conscious mental attitude by learning to think and to develop a relaxed brain.

1- Learning to think and how to think. The development of the brain's two hemispheres is primordial. The right one lets new thoughts, imagination, intuition, dreams, direct experiments, harmonious relations spurt out. The left one organizes them, structures them, manages them, administers them, analyzes them, puts them into words and calculates. In most people, the right brain is developed to about 20% of its capacity and the left one to about 80%. So, as meditation helps to develop the right brain, it is an adequate method to help achieve balance in this matter.

2- Learning to develop a profoundly relaxed brain. When one is able to produce profoundly relaxed waves so that an equilibrium of the "two brains" is reached, the pineal and pituitary glands give the strength needed to open the spiritual eye (third eye); access to internal vision becomes successful. To reach it, one must devote oneself to it, embody it, and infuse the work with daily energy.

The question asked at the fourth meeting of the International Spiritual Psychiatry Association (Association internationale de psychiatrie spirituelle, A.I.P.S.) held in Paris in March 1996 was: " Could psychotherapy, psychoanalysis lead to spirituality ? " In Asia and in Chinese traditional medicine, this question has long been answered. Energy is considered as the vector which conveys the physical, emotional, mental and spiritual data of the human being. To intervene at one level or another will have an impact on the other levels. Meditation practices do in fact bring back memories, phantasms and repressed internal images. The Zen method says "let thoughts pass through as clouds and bring attention back to breathing by inner focus on "breathe in/breathe out ". On the other hand, psychoanalysis and the transpersonnal psychotherapy of Marc-Alain Deschamps, are saying " confront phantasms within reality in order to free oneself from them" (Senk, 1996). In this last perspective, the patient becomes a warrior who confronts his inner world instead of utilizing it in a magical way.

Both Zen and Tao are saying the same thing: Sit down within the pain, don't run away from it, go through the pain and identify it, but also observe it as from a distance... without judgment, and let it " pass through as a cloud ". In order to reach the inner dimension where the self doesn't exist, it is necessary to distance oneself from the self, from the " image " we have of ourselves, from our injured and damaged image. It is necessary to renounce the ego, in order to create an opening and allow a second birth, on the plane of energy.

Three levels of meditation

We can reconized three levels ofTaoist meditation:

1. Physical: breathing and concentration on emotions and sensations, " Being in what is".
2. Mental: the silence of the thoughts, getting out of duality and contradiction.
3. Spiritual: spiritual awakening, access to pure intelligence, to healing and to natural laws.

Those three levels of meditation which aim at perfecting physical, psychological and spiritual health, are one and only one thing when looked at from the point of view of energy. Energy is neither good nor bad, it is neither physical, mental nor spiritual. It is always the same energy manifesting in different forms and in different ways. The mind form of energy is vitally important because, as a classical Chinese aphorism says, " the mind directs energy, energy directs the blood, and blood heals ". This is why the human being who has mental strength (Shen spiritual) can give to energy an impulsion, an orientation, a quality, a virtue which enables it to act on substance, on the blood (Xue). This is why physical and psychological approaches in Asia give such importance to meditation. In Chinese medicine, physical exercices are practiced together with breathing and circulation of energies, as in Qi Cong, which means the mastery (Cong) of energy (Qi). The Su Wen Nei Jing, ancient medical Chinese writings, are clearly saying that " acupuncture is for the ignorant ", meaning it is for those who have not learned to master Qi, either by practicing Qi Cong or meditation, and thus must have an external help (acupuncturist or doctor) to heal their being.

Qi Cong or mastery of the Qi, has different stages: sitting meditation, standing meditation or motion (Taï Chi) meditation; one must be able to meditate in all kinds of circumstances in order to reach the meditation state. With more advanced practices one reaches illumination by exiting the physical body to create the energy body (light body); this in turn strenghtens the subtle and spiritual bodies (crystal body), which can reinfuse the physical body.

Meditation is used to acquire knowledge of oneself as subject and object of the experiment. Self knowledge allows one to reach harmony, equilibrium, evolution of one's being, to acquire consciousness of one's internal dimension (the one that underlies substance) i.e. one's energy. During meditation thoughts come out of the subconscious or the unconscious; they appear on the screen of consciousness which contemplates them with indifference, as from a distance, and lets them disappear as ghosts from the past which have no hold on the present moment.

Threefold view of man

Freud developed the concepts of Ego, Id, SuperEgo and the unconscious, but he forgot the subconscious or supraconscious, which were more developed by Jung. Taoïst thinking removes the polemics of the Ego, Id, SuperEgo, and the opposition of consciousness to the unconsciousness. The Taoïst view , like the Christian , speaks of a three way view of man as BODY, MIND, and SPIRIT.
BODY: Jing and Qi: physical substance, sexuality;
MIND: Shen of the Heart: sensations, emotions, dualistic thinking, energy (Qi);
SPIRIT: Shen of the Soul: psychical activities, relative thinking, spirit.
Transitions from the physical level to the mind and energy level, and from the energy level to the spiritual level require each time a new birth, to "be born again".

The therapist can work at different levels - body - mind or spirit - only if he has walked and explored these paths himself. Jung spoke of alchemical proceedings; Taoïst meditation speaks of transformation. Magic is the realm of transformation. It works not through interference but through benevolent neutrality, through acting without acting, through speaking without words, guiding without guiding. These characteristics are possible because energy works on another level, away from matter and duality. Warriorship is the realm of the internal combat: "To confront our phantasms within reality ". It is this opposition from the ego which is the biggest obstacle to healing because it has a limited point of view and clings to the known, to the past, the old conditionings and to the recurrent schemes.

Meditation: sexuality, energy and spirituality

In cognitive therapy, sexuality tends to be excluded, as in religion and studied in the separate field of sexology. Instead, Taoists explain the link between sexuality (Jing Qi), food-emotions (Qi) and spirit (Shen). All three are treated in continuity, preserving the essence of life (sperms and ovaries) as a sacred process which creates an amplification and regeneration of organs and glands.

A circle around the body represents the "little celestial cycle" that Master Mantak Chia calls the "Microcosmic Orbit". This orbit empowers the human being to conserve his or her vital essence (JING), to transform it into energy (Qi) and mental (Shen), and to increase spiritual power. Sexual strenght in not denied or sublimated; it is used to spiritualize the person by the process of transformation through the points of energy of the Microcosmic Orbit and enhance with positive emotions.

Sexuality is not a purely physical or driven action but a conscious activity which can increase the energy born from positive emotions and transform it into mental and spiritual energy. When sexuality is peaceful, under the control of the mind and when a man knows how to " bring up the white tiger " which means to stop ejaculation; when a woman knows how to " master the red dragon " meaning to stop menstruation, when emotions are positive and harmonious, under the control of the mind, when the partners know how to " bring up the green dragon ", meaning they can master their emotions and have sexual intercourse which recharges the vital essence and brings it to a mind that becomes luminous, then the wise can sit down in peace and live within the present, within reality.

For the Taoists, man is responsible for his illness and " if one can make oneself ill, one can heal oneself " The load of negative emotions is used as a ground-source for one's positive energy. Pure light, the source of life, is always available, as seven rays of the rainbow. One of the goals ofTaoïst meditation is teaching the exterior sense organs to serve the emotions and the inner organs. These in turn relate to the luminous world and can recharge the vital essence through saliva and sexuality.

The sense organs and the body organs are the sources of sensations and emotions. For the Taoists, our five organs (lungs, kidneys, liver, heart and spleen) are considered as the sources of our energies. These energies can be negative or positive. It is still energy, transformable, changeable, with a conscious mind. Negative emotions affect organs and glands, making them stressed and sick, and in turn producing psychosomatic illness. Through consciousness, humans have the power to transform these negative emotions (sadness, fear, anger, hastiness and worry) and illness into positive emotions (courage, gentleness, kindness, love and openness) and health. Positive emotions combined together give the ability, through insight and the energy of good feelings, to practice forgiveness that is not induced solely by the mind nor from ideas or good intentions.

The same thing applies with regard to compassion. Taoïsts not only speak or think about compassion, they cultivate it, have it in all their cells, feel it inside themselves and act and speak with compassion. How do they cultivate compassion? They transform the five negative emotions into five positive emotions and add to those the sexual love energy or the vital essence to amplify the good energy of positive emotions and to experiment and feel compassion.

FIVE NEGATIVE EMOTIONS -- FIVE POSITIVE EMOTIONS = FORGIVENESS
FIVE NEGATIVE EMOTIONS -- FIVE POSIVITE EMOTIONS X SEX = COMPASSION

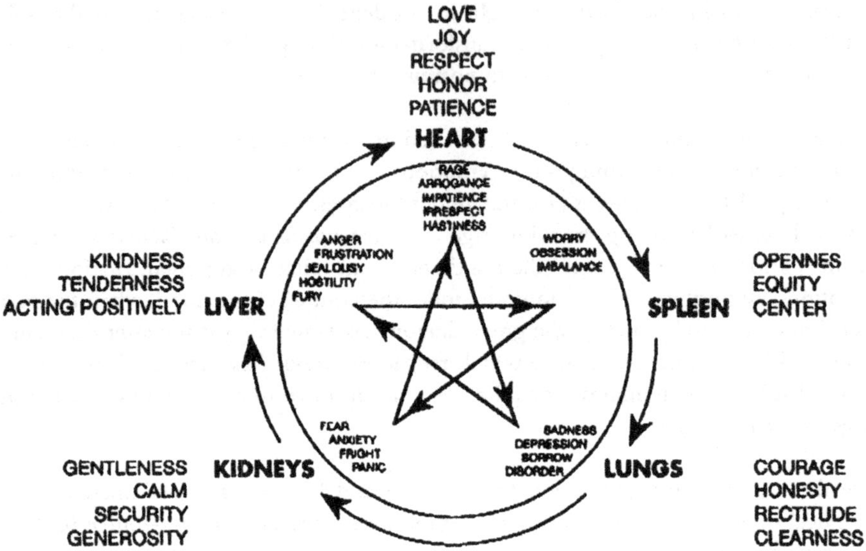

Figure 1. Transformation of negative emotions into positive emotions in taoïst meditation.

These good energies can be transformed and preserved within the body, in all points of the Microcosmic Orbit that recharges all seven glands and the five major organs, thus activating energy circulation by breathing in those points, protecting matter from sickness. (See Figure I).

"In fact, the elders obtained longevity through the seminal energy present in their bodies" (Lu Tson, 1969).
"Preserving the semen, transforming it into energy and recreating the physical body, energy and mind through the backward course "Microcosmic Orbit", such is the way of the Taoist saints and wisemen" (Lu Tsou, 1969).

Occidental therapists often consider emotions, sensations and sexual ejaculation as ends in themselves. This is why they work on going back into the past and very often forget the present. Oriental therapists consider emotions, sensations and vital essence as sources of spiritual energy, to be like "a fish in the water", a microcosm within a macrocosm, in the present and the future.

With the Taoist approach, happiness originates from forgiveness and compassion, themselves being born by a combination of the five positives emotions of the five organs: joy and love of the heart, lucidity and courage of the lungs, kindness and tenderness of the liver, openness and balance of the spleen, gentleness and quietness of the kidneys, preservation and spiritualization of the vital essence. Regarding sexual energy and the practice of meditation, adepts transfer sexual energy to the brain, thus " bringing the golden flower to the sinciput (top of the head) " (Lu Tsou, 1969) and back into the glands and organs. This results in harmonizing emotions into compassion and allows one to live on physical, mental and spiritual levels together. "The saints and the Wise-men have no other way of cultivating their life than to destroy sensual pleasure and preserve semen. This through the "backward course" of the "wheel of the back river" (Lu Tsou, 1969).

Man and woman reunited within ourselves: no more separation, no more surrender, but the feeling of being reunited with our masculine (Yang) (Fire) Li, and feminine (Yin) (Water) Kan, sides and with the universe. This is the way to reach individuation and the self that Jung speaks of. Being centered on oneself, enlightened, linked and balanced: this is the result of meditating upon oneself.

Meditation and psychotherapy: access to self healing

For a therapist, the goal of Taoïst meditation is to help people become responsible for themselves and to teach them how to heal themselves: " It is better to teach how to fish than to gives fishes ". At the same time, through the practice of directing energy through thought, one is able to help without words, and can listen more easily. The person arrives, speaks of her suffering, sadness, anger, obsession and fears. Taoist meditation practiced on others allows the therapist to bring to the person the light she needs, transmitting it to her from a close or a far distance and pacing according to emotion and attitude changes. To help in this matter, a knowledge of acupuncture is helpful. It is necessary to be able to practice " psychopuncture ", or autohypnosis, or the awakening of energy (Energetic Hypnosis) on a specific acupuncture point or organ, or the use of Qi Cong to obtain a healing effect. Taoist meditation also requires the theory of correspondences: the five elements, the six energies. (See Annex I: Chinese medicine correspondence charts - Human being). This knowledge allows one to choose the right suggestions, the right visualizations, the right acupuncture points to be toned up by the mind, and the Qi Cong exercises according to individual characteristics and syndrome types and to teach the patient to do the same for him or herself. A few examples of the integration of psychology, acupuncture, Qi Cong and meditation have been detailed in a conference - Psychology and Traditional Medicine: Using the mind to increase healing power and maximizing acupuncture treatments (Tremblay, 1993) and have been published later under the title: Psychology and Chinese Traditional Medicine. (Tremblay, 1994) Jeremy Ross, in his book " Acupuncture points combinations " specifies the same idea " [...] acupuncture can be readily combined with energy work and meditation." (Ross, 1995). The theory of hypnosis evolves in a similar pattern: awakening people instead of putting them to sleep. "Tear them away from the hypnosis of routine thoughts that make them robots and paralyze their abilities" and make them more self-reliant in the healing process: " it is the patient who hypnotizes himself and takes his suffering in charge" (Dehin, 1994).

Many people come to therapist with desires of happiness and well-being. But very often they reject the source of their happiness: i.e. their apparent misfortune, their seem-

Annex 1. Chinese medicine correspondence charts[1]

HUMAN BEING CORRESPONDENCES					
Mental	PRO	ZHI	HUN	SHEN	I
Position	Laying down	Standing up	Walking	Observating	Sitted
Expression	Sobbing	Trembling	Outcrying	Laughing	Singing
Voice	Peevish, tearful	Sigh, whine	Strong, high-pitched	Laughing	Singing
Character	Firm		Peaceful	Active	Quiet
Body liquid	Spittle	Urine	Tears	Sweat	Saliva
Negative emotions	Sadness	Fear	Anger	Hate	Obsession
Positive emotions	Courage	Sweetness	Goodness	Love	Opened
Reaction to changes	Cough	Shivers	Seizure	Sadness	Yellowish tint
Senses	Touch	Hearing	Seeing	Speaking	Taste
Senses organs	Nose	Ears	Eyes	Tongue	Mouth
Internal organs	Lungs	Kidneys	Liver	Heart	Spleen
Specific functions	Energy	Will, bones	Nerves	Blood	Flesh
Bowel	Large intestine	Bladder	Gall-bladder	Small intestine	Stomach
Texture	Skin, hair	Hairs, bones teeth	Muscle, nails vein, tendon	Artery, blood complexion	Flesh, lips mucous

ing ill-being. Instead they should explore and consider them as part of life, as a reality, like the two sides of the same coin, as life's paradox and an indefectible law. Happiness is the ability to welcome the pleasant without dwelling on it and receiving the unpleasant without condemning it. Constant happiness is an impossible goal in the material and emotional dualistic world. What makes pleasure possible is also the source of our miseries. Most people remain on a dual level of thinking, like white or black and have not achieved relative thinking which is white and black at the same time. Relative thinking is customary for the Asians as they are trained in the double complementary contradiction ofYin/Yang.

The search for pleasure, or joy, and or emotional satisfaction through the physical senses has no end. Nobody finds happiness in it because it leads to pleasure and displeasure just as the pleasure of erection-ejaculation leads to a post-orgasmic depression or " little death ". "The fool wastes the supreme jewel of his body in uncontrolled sensual pleasure and is unable to preserve his seminal energy. When it has thus reached its term, the body perishes" (Lu Tsou, 1996).

The law of relativity is everywhere just as the law of death is part of life. There is no permanence within living creatures. Unhappiness also comes because we see things from our own point of view, unable as we are to appreciate them as others around us do, or to rise above problems. Seeing and observing things not as a victim, or a culprit, or a judge but as an interested observer is the key. No matter what happens, what counts is the way of reacting to things and our attitude towards them.

Conclusion

In the end, Taoist masters worked on many techniques: relaxation, breathing, concentration, inspiration of light, solar energy and " assimilation of the lunar flower " in order to keep and reinforce vital energy.

According to Master Mantak Chia, it is possible to transform the negative effects of lack of energy or of energy blocks (closed or empty points) into positive effects, into active energy (open or full points) which sustains health and vitality. This is made possible through breathing and daily meditation on each point of the Microcosmic Orbit. The entire Taoïst system is based on the learning of breathing-visualizing-feeling the energy in the microcosmic orbit. This exercise is helpful in sitting meditation " sitting in peace ", in standing meditation with the Qi Cong, in the sexual exercises which keep the energy within the sperm and ovaries, in the Tai Ji exercise of breathing in the spine and projecting energy to the hands. It is also useful in the martial arts. These exercises heal different illnesses but also make the adepts of martial and other arts more alert, more dynamic and more able to progress rapidly, because they are less tired and less in need of sleep. They have more vigor and vitality.

The Taoïst meditation method of" sitting in peace " brings peace to the mind, restores health and develops inner harmonization. It is widely practised in Asia." It consists of a non-sectarian way of reaching mental quietness, regardless of any religion or religious ritual." This is very important in order to avoid any kind of polemic. The Taoist meditation is a way to liberate whatever hinders the intellect, health and the laws of nature in ourselves. The Taoist concept follows the models set by nature. Master Chia said : As our energy body, our energetic network is part of ourselves, all these Taoist exercises help us discover and feel the Qi as part of the human continuum: i.e. the energy of one's body, of other bodies, of nature all around us.

References

Aung, Steven, (1995). *Revue Française de Médecine Traditionnelle Chinoise, no. 168*, p. 203-207.

Bichen, Zhao, (1979). *Traite d'alchimie et de physiologie taoïste,* trad. Despeux, C., Les deux Océans, Paris, 193 pages.

Chamfrault, A., (1981). *Traité de médecine chinoise: Les livres sacrés de médecine chinoise* -Tome 2 - Editions Chamfrault, Angouleme, 575 pages.

Chia, Mantak, (1983). *Awaken Healing Energy through the Tao,* Aurora Press, Santa Fe, 193 pages.

Chia, Mantak, (1991). *Fusion des cinq Élèments: Méditations fondamentales et avancées pour transformer les Émotions négatives,* Paris, Guy Trédaniel Editeur, 203 pages.

Dehin, Robert, (1994) *La Nouvelle Hypnose. Elle n'endort pas elle réveille!* Guide Ressources, Montréal, November, Vol. 10, no.3.

Edde, Gérard, (1988).. *Méditation et Santé, selon les traditions et les médecines chinoises,* Albin Michel, spiritualité vivante, 209 pages.

Krisnamurti, (1987). *La Flamme de l'Attention,* Editions du Rocher, Paris.

Lao, Tseu, (1967). *Tao To King,* idées Gallimard, Trad. du livre Kia Hway, 188 pages.

Lu, Tsou, (1969) *Le Secret de la Fleur d'Or*, Librairie Mèdicis, Paris, 143 pages.

Ross, Jeremy, (1995.) *Acupuncture Points Combination*, Ed. Churchill, Levingstone, 476 pages.

Senk, Pascale, (1996). *Psychologies, Ame et psyché: dialogues au sommet*, no 143, pp. 62-65.

Tremblay, Nicole, (1994). *Revue Française de Médecine traditionnelle chinoise*, Psychologie et Médecine traditionnelle chinoise, no.164, pp.170-181.

Tremblay, Nicole, (1990). La continuité par la théorie et la pratique des correspondances exprimées par les symboles graphiques et ontologiques. Thèse de doctorat, *La Symbolique dans la Médecine Traditionnelle Chinoise.* Université Laval.

Tremblay, Nicole, (1988). L'Orbite Microcosmique ou le petit cycle cosmique, consolidation, traduction et commentaires des notes et des livres de Maótre Mantak Chia - Quèbec, 42 p. (brochure non publiée)

Van Nghi, Ngugen, (1989). *Art et Pratique de l'Acupuncture et de la Moxibustion selon Zhen Jiu Da Chang,* Tome II-III, Editions N.V.N.

Krishnamurti, (1987). *La flamme de l'attention,* Paris, Points, Ed. du Rocher, p. 154

Senk, P. (1966). Ame et psyché; dialogues au sommet, *Psychologies*, 143, p. 62.

Senk, P. (1966). *Amet psyché;* dialogues au sommet, Psychologies, 143, p.62.

Tremblay, N. (1994). *Revue Française de Médecine traditionnelle chinoise,* Psychologie et Médecine Traditionnelle Chinoise, no. 164, pp. 170-181.

Chia, M. (1983). *Awaken Healing Energy Through the Tao,* Aurora Press, Santa Fé, p. 32, digram 11.

Lu Tsou, (1969). *Le secret de la fleur d'or.*, Librairie Médicis, Paris, p.118

Idem, p.119.

Idem, p. 11.

Idem, p.119.

Given by the author in November 1993, at a seminar of the Association of Acupunctorists registered at the C.P.M.Q., Montréal.

Tremblay, N. (1994). Psychologie et médecine traditionnelle chinoise, *Revue Française de Médecine Traditionnelle Chinoise,* no 164, pp. 170-182.

Ross, J. (1995). Acupuncture Points Combination, Ed. Churchill Levingstone, p.5.

Dehin, R. (1994). La nouvelle Hypnose. Elle n'endort plus, elle réveille! *Guide Ressources,* 10, pp. 27-28.

Lu Tsou, (1969). *Le secret de la fleur d'or,* Librairie Médicis, Paris, pp. 118-119.

Edde, G. (1988). *Méditation et Santé, selon les Traditions et les Médecines Chinoises,* Albin Michel,spiritualité vivante, pp. 134.

Tremblay, N. (1990). La continuité par la théorie et la pratique des correspondances exprimées par les symboles graphiques et ontologiques, Thése de Doctorat, Université Laval, pp. 19 to 28.

THE PRIMACY OF MIND IN EARLY BUDDHIST PSYCHOLOGY

Padmal de Silva,
Senior Lecturer and Consultant Clinical Psychologist, Department of Psychology, Institute of Psychiatry, University of London.

Résume

This paper discusses the place of mind in the psychology of Early, or Therav da, Buddhism. Canonical and commentarial texts are examined in order to elucidate this. The primacy of mind is a key feature in Buddhist psychology, and the paper discusses the significance of this in Buddhism. Special attention is paid to the areas of personal development and behavioural change. The role of mind in one's endeavours in these directions is discussed. In the discussion, several relevant terms and concepts in Early Buddhism are also examined in some detail.

Introduction

In this paper, a major aspect of Buddhist psychology will be discussed - namely, the central place accorded to mind. This is an aspect of Buddhist psychology that some may see as self-evident, yet it is not always fully appreciated, and even scholars who are in agreement with this position often neglect the significance of it in the overall framework of Buddhist psychology.

First, a general introductory point. This paper limits its discussion to Early Buddhism. By the term 'Early Buddhism', I mean Theravàda Buddhism, which is the form of Buddhism that is contained in the early Pali language texts. While there are many significant areas of overlap between Theravàda Buddhism and later schools, the former is considered to be the most loyal representation of the original teachings of the Buddha. The literature of Early Buddhism consists of:

(a) the original Buddhist canon put together soon after the Buddha's death and committed to writing in the first century of the Christian Era;

(b) the early commentaries in the Pali language which were in their present form by the end of the first century of the Christian Era (e.g. *Sumangalavilàsini*), and

(c) other Pali texts of the same time period which may be described as expository and/or interpretive works (e.g. *Visuddhimagga*).

The canon itself is comprised of three parts: the *Sutta Pitaka*, which contains the discourses of the Buddha on various occasions; the *Vinaya Pitaka*, which contains the rules of discipline to monks and nuns; and the *Abhidhamma Pitaka*, which contains highly systematized philosophical and psychological analyses, which were finalised into their current form about 250 B.C. - i.e., later than the material in the other two parts.

The books of the canon are listed in Table I.

TABLE I Individual Books of the Buddhist Canon

Sutta Pitaka
- *Digha Nikàya*
- *Majjhima Nikàya*
- *Sanyutta Nikàya*
- *Anguttara Nikàya*
- *Khuddaka Nikàya*

Vinaya Pitaka
- *P timokkha*
- *Khandhaka*
- *Nikàya*

Abhidhamma Pitaka
- *Dhammasangani*
- *Vibhanga*
- *Dhàtukathà*
- *Puggalapaññatti*
- *Kathàvatthu*
- *Yamaka*
- *Patthàna*

Mind in Early Buddhism

Key terms:
It is necessary to consider, at this point, the terminology of Early Buddhism in relation to mind and mental phenomena. There are several key terms, which are overlapping and inter-related. The main ones are *citta, mano* and *viññàna*. In several instances, the three are treated synonymously, but an examination of the literature illuminates their different shades of meaning. Several discussions of these terms are available in the literature, including an influential early paper by Johansson (1965).

Citta is used, in its most general sense, to refer to the invisible and uncorporeal energiser of the body and as the activator of the personality. The term is usually translated as 'mind'. It is described as a series of events in an incessant process of mentation. In the worldly individual (i.e., one also has not attained perfection), it is seen as 'throbbing and wavering'. It 'travels far, fares alone, is uncorporeal, and resident in a cave - i.e. concealed'. It is often 'frightened, agitated, alarmed and flushed'. In the worldly individual, it is afflicted with immoral needs and emotions.

The pre-eminent function of *citta*, in relation to the worldly individual and his world, consists in its ideological leadership. In the words of the Buddha, 'the world is led by *citta*, is swept away by *citta*; the world comes under the power of *citta*'.

Citta is, in its original nature, pure and resplendent. How is it corrupted, as it is found in worldly beings? It is corrupted by defilements (*upakkilesa*). These defilements are not an integral part of *citta*. The defilements include: excitement of sensual pleasure, malevolence, sloth and torpor, agitation and worry, and perplexity. These are considered hindrances to one's personal and moral development.

The second relevant term is *mano*. *Mano* is seen as the intellectual function of consciousness. Perhaps it is best understood, following the analysis of David Kalupahana (1987), in the context of the Buddhist account of perception and cognition. Perception is based on the twelve gateways (*àyatana*), six of these being the five sense organs plus *mano*, which may be seen as an inner sense, and the other six being the objects of these. The status of *mano* is special, as it has the ability to reflect on the objects of the other senses. Kalupahana points out that its function is to assist in bringing back the impressions produced by the other sense faculties, and as such constitutes a form of reflection. *Mano* therefore has concepts (*dhammà*) as its objects, and these are generally considered substitutes for percepts. This reflective faculty also contributes to the sense of personal identity or the conception of self.

Table 2 provides an illustration of this analysis of perception and cognition.

TABLE 2 The Factors Involved in Cognition

Sense Organ	Object	Consciousness
eye	material shapes	visual consciousness
ear	sounds	auditory consciousness
nose	smells	olfactory consciousness
tongue	tastes	gustatory consciousness
body	tangibles	tactile consciousness
mind	mental objects	mental consciousness

It will have been noted that Table 2 above refers to consciousness, which leads us to the other main term which needs discussion. This is *viññàna*. Its translation as `consciousness' is almost universal amongst Buddhist scholars. *Viññàna* may be seen as ego-consciousness; however, in contrast to the Upanisadic view that consciousness (*vijñaàa*) is representative of an eternal and unchanging soul or self (*àtman*), the Buddhist concept refers to a conditioned event, arising from other factors. The Buddhist notion of a stream of consciousness (*viññàna-sota*) is very similar to the view of William James on this subject and helps one to understand what *viññana* means.

A further concept which merits consideration, if only for the sake of completeness, is that of *cetanà*. This term, commonly found in the texts, refers to the 'willing' or 'motivational' function of mental activity. The term has been variously translated as will, volition, effort, aspiration, intention and purpose, among others. In a much-cited passage, the Buddha says: "Monks, I declare *cetan* to be moral action (*kamma*)". The sense of will, involving choice, is paramount here. The term is extensively analysed in the expository literature. In the *Visuddhimagga*, Buddhaghosa distinguishes between four types of *cetanà*: (i) volitions impelling the individual from within himself; (ii) volitions induced within the individual by others prevailing on him; (iii) volitions operating within the individual with his knowledge that they do so; and (iv) volitions that operate with no such knowledge. The final category, it appears, refers to unconscious motivation.

The power of the mind:

It was noted earlier how the mind, mostly described by the term *citta*, is a powerful force that leads the individual to action. The worldly person is governed and led by his mind - by his mind which is contaminated by various defilements. In Early Buddhism, one is asked to strive to have the mind under control, and it is explicitly stated that the mind can be brought under control.

The *Dhammapada*, which is part of the *Khuddaka Nikàya* of the *Sutta Pitaka*, has several clear, pithy statements which reflect this. To cite a few:

'Phenomena have mind at their pre-condition, are dominated by the mind, and are mind-made'.

'As rain penetrates a badly-thatched house, so does lust penetrate an uncultivated mind'.

'As rain does not penetrate a well-thatched house, so lust does not penetrate a well-cultivated mind'.

'A wise man strenghtens his trembling and wavering mind, which is difficult to guard and hard to check, even as a fletcher strengtens an arrow'.

'Beneficial is the restraining of mind that is difficult to restrain, which is fleeting and wandering at will; a restrained mind is a bringer of happiness'.

'Neither one's mother nor one's father, nor other relatives will do much; a rightly directed mind will do one greater service'.

It is through the control of mind that the individual controls his life and moves towards personal and moral development. Professor O. H. de A. Wijesekera referred to this aspect of Buddhist psychology, in a paper published over thirty years ago, as its 'great optimism' (Wijesekera, 1961). The defilements can be got rid of, and the mind can be controlled by the mind itself (*cetasà cittam abhinigganhàti*. It is said that the mind, when properly cultivated, is the most pliable thing to handle (*kammaniya*). What, one might ask, is this cultivation? The answer, in Buddhist psychology, is a very clear one. The cultivation of mind is, of course, *bhàvanà*. This Pali word is today commonly translated as 'meditation', but etymologically it means 'cultivation' or 'development'.

It has been previously pointed out by many, including the persent author, that Buddhist meditation (I use the word here to mean *bhàvanà*) provides a potent means of personal and moral development (see de Silva, 1986). This endeavour, using several techniques, has been claimed to lead to major changes in one's conduct, behaviour, and cognitions. In the classical religious sense, meditation techniques can lead to a personal and moral transformation of the person. This is the state of being on *arahant* (`worthy one' or `perfect one'). In this state one perceives the world without distortions caused by defilements of any kind. One's perception is free, and direct appraisal of objects becomes not just possible but also the norm. What else does the *arahant* state entail? In one description, it is said:

'The *arahant* has destroyed the cankers, lived the life, done what needed to be done, achieved well-being, shattered life's fetters, and is freed by perfect knowledge. He has applied himself to six things - dispassion, detachment, harmlessness, destruction of craving, destruction of grasping, and non-delusion'.

The *arahant's* actions do not emanate from the common sources of passion (*lobha*), hatred (*dosa*) and delusion (*moha*), which are the springs of behaviour of wordly beings. He is, however, capable of joy, or positive sentiment. He has loving kindness (*mett*) to all, and he has compassion (*karunà*). The *arahant's* life is also characterised by nine standards of behaviour. He can not and does not engage in: taking of life, stealing, sexual contact, uttering falsehoods, enjoying the comforts of wealth, and going astray through desire, through hate, through delusion, and through fear. It is also said that such behaviours are 'endenburgimpossibilities'. The *arahant's* life is also characterised by alertness; it is said he is incapable of carelessness (*pamàda*).

While the cultivation of mind can thus, in the ultimate analysis, lead to personal and moral development amounting to a transformation of the person, it also leads to many other tangible, more mundane, benefits. In fact, for the lay person who has not totally renounced his ordinary life in a quest for the *arahant* state, meditation can produce other benefits. These, in the accounts given in Early Buddhist texts, include the following: calmness, greater ability to concentrate, greater freedom from distractions, control of unwholesome desires, greater tolerance of change and turmoil around oneself, sharper awareness of one's own responses, ability to achieve restful sleep, and the control of pain.

There is no need, in this paper, to cite the substantial evidence available in modern psychology and psychiatry which shows that the claims made in Early Buddhism for the benefits of meditation are indeed supportable. Particularly impressive is the work on pain control (cf. Kabat-Zinn, Lipworth and Burney, 1985), one area specifically described in the texts on more than one occasion. I have discussed the parallels between the Early Buddhist references to, and theories of, pain control through meditation and the theories and findings of present-day clinical research in previous communications (see de Silva, 1990), so I shall not dwell on them here.

Mind and the Path towards Development

Some comments are now in order on the way towards personal and spiritual development, the Noble Eightfold Path. This is the way (*magga*), the fourth of the Four Noble Truths, which is a fundamental teaching in Buddhism. The way consists of eight aspects:

(i) right view
(ii) right thought
(iii) right speech
(iv) right action
(v) right livelihood
(vi) right effort
(vii) right mindfulness, and
(viii) right concentration.

This list contains five elements which are essentially mental, emphasizing once again the high place accorded to the mind in personal and moral development. The final two in the list, midfulness and concentration, are the crucial elements in meditation, which we have discussed earlier. While all the eight elements are important parts of the path, it is these two that enable one to make the final transition to a transformed state.

An alternative account of the scheme of personal and moral development is also found in Early Buddhism. This is the three-fold scheme of training. The three aspects here are:

(i) restraint in conduct (*śila*),
(ii) concentration (*samàdhi*), and
(iii) insight (*paññà*).

These three are seen as progressive and mutually dependent. While restraint is a necessary pre-condition, the other two, which are both essentially mind-based, are crucial for the attainment of moral perfection.

Thus, it is clear that while Early Buddhism does not negate the importance of behavioural change (restraint) in one's quest for development, the pride of place is accorded to the psychological factors. Furthermore, even behavioural and verbal restraint is considered as a necessary first step in the overall psychological development and effort that is needed. Practice of restraint is the method by which one could be vigilant about one's overt behaviours; this is done through abstention and conscious self-control, and the practice of the opposite (to immoral) types of actions. This enables a transformation to occur at the grossest and most tangible level. In concentration, an attempt is made to bring about focus and composure to the mind, in order to prevent the excitement of unwholesome emotions. Here, one takes full conscious control of one's mental activity. This enables the elimination, at least temporarily, of certain unwholesome emotions, and the development of certain wholesome emotions such as compassion and equanimity. Insight is believed to deal with the moral evil at the very source. This is the understanding that eradicates all sources of immorality in a way that they are not revived again. Ignorance of the true nature of things is eliminated. The attainment of the final emancipating knowledge is the peak of moral development. This is, in essence, an achievement of the mind, by the mind, and through the mind.

References

de Silva, P. (1986). Buddhism and behaviour change: Implications for therapy. In: G. Claxton (Ed.) *Beyond Therapy: The Impact of Eastern Religions on Psychological Theory and Practice*, London: Wisdom.

de Silva, P. (1990). Buddhist psychology: A review of theory and practice, *Current Psychology: Research and Reviews*, **9**, 236-254.

Johansson, R. E. A. (1965). Citta, mano, viññàa: A psychosemantic investigation, *University of Ceylon Review*, **23**, 165-215.

Kabat-Zinn, J., Lipworth, L. and Burney, R. (1985). The clinical use of mindfulness meditation for the self-regulation of chronic pain, *Journal of Behavioural Medicine*, **8**, 163-190.

Kalupahana, D. J. (1987). *The Principles of Buddhist Psychology*, Albany: State University of New York Press.

Wijesekera, O. H. de A. (1961). *The Buddhist Concept of Mind*, Bodhi Leaves, No. A.9, Kandy: Buddhist Publication Society.

Note: The Canonical texts have all been published by the Pali Text Society in London. They are also available in English translations, again published by the same body. The same applies to the two non-Canonical works referred to in this paper, *Sumangalavilàsini* and *Visuddhimagga*.

MIND AND BODY: DUALISTIC NOTION OF NON-DUALISTIC NATURE: ISSUES FOR THE SCIENTIST - PRACTITIONER

Saroja Srinivasan, M.A.,D.A.P.(Clin)., Ph.D.,
Clinical Psychologist, PSYCNET Psychology Consultant, Sydney, Australia

These last two days we have journeyed through exciting unchartered waters experiencing a connection within ourselves and outside of ourselves. It is truly an experience that would be hard to describe in words. Yet the fact that we have experienced it brings forward the very subject matter of our symposium " mind and body". Our presence here is testimony to the interface between the two. We come from diverse geographical, cultural and other "physical" backgrounds and as professionals with our diverse epistemological positions which are surely 'mental' constructs. Life as a conscious human being is surely a combination of both body and mind each equally necessary for the other. A body without the functioning mind is a corpse and a mind without the functioning body is an intangible soul. As Hodgson (1991) puts it "Apart from the mind, external reality may be considered as little more than a cosmic code" (P.188).

The title of this paper was chosen for two reasons. (a) The term 'scientist-practitioner' is often used in training programs in clinical psychology. Exactly what brand of science is hardly specified, thus leading to a variety of approaches. Techniques are addressed that stem from different models yet they are often evaluated on the basis of the prevailing paradigm of the academic department. (b) Because a number of these techniques originate from philosophies based on different epistemologies, they warrant a different methodology for their evaluation. It is possible that often what we have is 'science on the cheap' as Sheldrake(1994) points out. In this paper I would like to explore the non-dualistic approach to mind-body questions as it affects a clinician.

Charles Hendel, Emeritus Professor of Philosophy and Metaphysics at Yale University, more than 20 years ago, wrote in the forward to Wilber Penfield's "Mystery of the mind" (1975) : "The philosophy of the day must concern itself about the actual facts of the day's experience or it becomes useless and irreleveant. There is little profit in trying to formulate "the problem of mind and body" and then relate the present 'wonder' about the mind to the answer to that old question .... we must reckon with the evidence and experiments of today and find their position accordingly." (p.xxii).

To try and answer the question posed for our seminar in the light of the above quote is indeed a formidable task in the 1990s. Where do we look for the evidence and experiments? Do we look to neurologists and neurosurgeons such as Penfield and many others before him dating back to the 1800s and the phrenology movements or perhaps even earlier to Leonardo da Vinci during the renaissance? Do we look to the evidence gathered by experts in the field of mathematics and physics and chemistry who supply us with powerful 4arguments for the physical basis of life or do we look to the impetus

derived from additions from professionals such as computer scientists and cognitive scientists? Of course this list of experts is incomplete without the inclusion of philosophers who have pondered over this mind-matter, mind-body question for centuries without a clear consensus. Added to this of course are the socio-political theories which have influenced the models of mind that are expounded. At no time, as in the last twenty-five years, has there been more interest in understanding the relationship between mind and body/matter. Early this century, Sir Charles Sherrington, eminent physiologist and Nobel prize winner, said "Mind, meaning by that thoughts, memory, feelings, reasoning and so on , is difficult to bring into a class of physical things".
John Locke queried more than 300 years ago, "How do we separate imagination and madness?". We are no closer to answering many questions. Within the constraints posed by a 'scientific' mode of enquiry that is based on the prevailing paradigm, questions such as the following are still debated: What is the brain action that makes the distinction possible between these two aspects of mental behaviour? What is the reason and mechanism for the convincing kaleidoscopic activities of our dreams? How do we explain hypnosis or pain relief with acupuncture? What is the relation of mind to our many varieties of 5religious experience? How does the brain-mind construct a coherent self and world?
The focus of the arguments presented in trying to answer the above questions invariably reflects the particular slant of the prevailing paradigm. There are numerous dilemmas faced by a clinician when working under the assumptions of the prevailing paradigm which in itself is clouded with divergent models and methodologies despite stemming from the same epistemological foundation. Here the term 'science' is itself seen as being multifaceted. For example, one may cater to the inductive/empirical method or follow Popper's falsification approach or as mentioned earlier choose to use the prevailing paradigm approach. Page (1996) describes the various approaches and compares the fragmentation within clinical psychology practice to the experiences of a 'multiple personality" based on such divergent models of science.

Most clinicians, I would suggest, tend to be paradigmatic in their adherence to the scientific model. The prevailing paradigm for this scientific-practice of clinical psychology, is very much inductive, experimental with emphasis on collection of observable tangible data in a mechanistic reductionist framework. In clinical practice, the data one collects are not only what is observed by the clinician but also experiential data presented by the patient or client. Whilst it may be difficult to verify this data, their authenticity cannot be ignored. Within the model under which a clinician functions, "acceptable" data are almost always at the molecular and sub-molecular level, yet what the clinician is presented with is a gross manifestation of the mind-body phenomenon in all its subtelty, in the form of a feeling-thinking being who happens at this time to have a need to make things better or feel more happy or be pain-free or improve relationships or whatever may be important at present. As a practitioner, the most important task is to mobilise the client/patient to move from despair to hope, from anxiety to calmness. As a scientist, one is faced with the many faces of science, each with its own definitionsof what science should be. Most scientist-practitioners are looking to practice a personalised science and not a de-humanised science. Many variations on the same theme of what the scientific model is as well as many themes are still prevalent. Be it inductive, empiricist, falsificationist or 'anarchist' , there is no clear consensus among psychologists as to what is acceptable as a methodology for researching the efficacy of various techniques. As Page (op cit) says "While each of the clinicians .... are scientist - practitioners, the philosophies of science lead them to choose and evaluate theories and treatments in different ways" (P105). This is within the western-scientific arena. If one were to approach it from the eastern-experiential model, it would be even more complex, for the assumptions on which the approaches are based are entirely different.

The Yoga-Vedantatradition sees mind and body as essentially being two sides of a coin. The entire creation is seen on the basis of non-duality. Mind and matter are seen as phenomena that are two aspects of the same. The bi-directional interaction between the mind and body is acknowledged. Since knowledge is based on the interplay between contrasts and opposites, the contrasting that is needed to understand this 'oneness' of mind and matter is available only when we have experienced 'no-mind' and 'no-matter'. This is the goal of the pursuit of knowlwedge, in this tradition, and various methods are elucidated to achieve it .The techniques of quiet contemplation with the mind are encouraged to gain a thorough understanding.
As a clinician , when I am faced with the challenge of helping an individual make sense of his or her world and help them find what seems an elusive state of 'happy-being', I find myself increasingly presenting an integrated approach that addresses the interactive nature of mind and body. The traditional model of the Indian Ayurvedic approach, for example, stems from a theory of mind and body. This model sees human beings as not just machines that have learned to think but suggests that how and what we think affects our body and how we treat our body affects our mental prowess. This approach sees biology and psychology as far more closely intertwined than how it is seen in the western 'scientific' view.

If we can accept that the mind and body are integrated and are only two kinds of manifestations of the same energy we begin to perceive and experience everything quite differently. Such an integrated approach demands of individuals a total shift in the way they perceive the world and even more so their own experience. The Vedantic approach to the alleviation of 'suffering' is indeed quite topical in the clinician's room. The methods that are espoused in the classical vedantic tradition are geared towards the aspect of suffering that stems from frustration and discontent. Here we are not talking of physical pain but suffering caused by a sense of lack of fulfilment experienced by a reasonably 'healthy' person. We are referring to the 'suffering' portrayed by the 'worried well'. Taking a non-dualistic approach, this suffering would be addressed by training the person to become aware of the somatic manifestations of the 'mental' constructs of 'suffering'. A prime example of this approach is given by Patanjali's Yoga sutras which amount to a masterly exposition of the science, philosophy and practice of the yoga technique. In the Buddhist tradition, the Vipassana meditation technique trains one to discern the subtlest of sensations within the body. With consistent practice, the connectedness between thoughts and sensations become clear. With repetition, one becomes aware of the connection between physical and thought-based reactions that maintain the state of 'suffering'.In this method, resolution has to happen at an experiential level.The role of the teacher is to set up 'experiments' for the experience of the connectedness between mind and body to occur.This may take the form of dialogues or the setting up of situations for experiential learning to occur.Within the supportive and safe confines of this unique relationship between teacher and student, the experiments in experiential learning come to fruition. Not only does this method address the interaction of the (mind and body, it also extends the temporal and spatial constructs that limit ordinary everyday experience. The yoga-vedanta approach helps to view the complexity of the mind-body interaction in all its complexity , from the perspectives of both the inner and existential and its more gross manifestation in the form of the body.

So, after this brief and rather general look at a profound subject matter, what we have, in the traditional wisdom traditions that are based on experiential knowledge, is a complex framework which encompasses not only epistemological issues such as the nature of reality, self, and inter-personal and trans-personal connections but also more conventional reality issues such as the mind-body relationship.In conclusion, as practitioners it is imperative that we take on B an intensive exploration of this 'mind and body' approach with its rich experiential data to further our scientific pursuits.

REFERENCES

Chopra, D. (1993). *Ageless Body, Timeless Mind*, Harmony Books, New York, U.S.A.

Hodgson, D.(1991). *The Mind Matters,* Clarendon Press, Oxford, United Kingdom.

Taimni, I.K. (1986). *The Science of Yoga* (7th edition), The Theosophical Publishing House, Adyar, India.

Page, C. (1996).The Scientist-Practitioner Model: More faces than Eve, *Australian Psychologist,* Vol.3, No. 2.

Penfield, W. (1975). *The Mystery of the Mind* , Princeton University Press, New Jersey, U.S.A.

Sacks, O. (1993). *An Anthropologist on Mars*, Picador, U.K.

Sheldrake, R. (1994) Prayer : A Challenge for Science, *Noetic Sciences Review* , No. 30.

STUDY OF THE PSYCHOLOGY AND THE BEHAVIORAL SCIENCE OF QIGONG

Dr. Weidong Wang,
China Academy of Traditional Chinese Medicine, Guang An Men Hospital

Chinese Qi-gong is therapeutically divided into external Qi-gong and internal Qi-gong. As a self-control method, internal Qi-gong is divided into dynamic Qi-gong and static Qi-gong. A variety of self--control methods have been devised through a combination of three factors; image and self-instruction, breathing and posture, and movement.

The image and self-instruction is basically the same as self-hypnotism, and it is, as a training method, comparable to the Chinese medicine and Qi-gong theory and it is believed to affect a human body through complex workings of the nervous system as dictated by the cerebral cortex. From this perspective, studies on the subject must be conducted with physiological and psychological aspects in mind.

The breathing method, as a way of Qi-gong training, is believed to affect human physiology and psychology through an adjustment of autonomic nerve functions. From this perspective, studies on the subject must be conducted with psychophysiological and behavioral aspects born in mind.

The Qi-gong posture and movement, which includes molar behavior and molecular behavior is believd to have a considerable effect on physiology and psychology, and here comes into the picture body psychology and behavioral theory as subjects of study.

External Qi-gong therapy is basically believed to be hypnotherapeutic. The relevant theory is comparable to that of Chinese medicine and general Qi-gong theory, and its practice is based on psychological and behavioral theory.

I CONCEPT AND CLASSIFICATION OF QIGONG

According to clinical practice, the Qigong exercise can be divided into "external Qigong" and "internal Qigong. External Qigong, as a therapy is applied by physicians or the distributors of Qi to treat patients; and internal Qigong is practiced by the patients themselves for treatment of their diseases and preserving their health. This is similar to the classification of hypnotism into the heterohypnotism and autohypnotism. The former is a therapy applied by the hypnotists and the latter is done by the practitioners themselves. It does not mean the Chinese Qigong therapy is completely same as the western hypno-therapy and the psychological and behavioral differences between them will be further discussed.

Qigong
- External Qigong
- Internal Qigong

Fig. 1. Classification of Qigong

For the practice of internal Qigong, the breath is adjusted and the physical exercise is performed controlling the thoughts of patients. Therefore, it may produce an effect on the mental and physical activities of the human body. Through changing the posture, adjusting the breath and concentrating the mind, the practice of internal Qigong exercise can improve the physical, respiratory and mental functions and regulate the psychological, physiological and locomotive activities to prevent and treat diseases, strengthen the physique, increase intelligence and prolong one's life span after the body and mind are successfully balanced and integrated and the physiological and psychological potential energy is effectively mobilized. There were many methods of Qigong practice mentioned in ancient Chinese literature, such as Daoyin (a method of physical and breathing exercise), Tuna (adjustment of breath), Liandan (motivation of active substances), and Shoushen, Cunxiang, Zuowang or Chanding (adjustment of mental activity). After the analysis, summarization and inference of countless methods of Qigong practice, the intrinsic essence of them and the internal relationships between them can be summed up as "3 important essentials of Qigong practice", namely posture, breath and mental concentration, instead of 1 word Qi. The Qigong exercises of different academic schools, or different variations, may be divided into the following types according to the particular emphasis on any one of the 3 important essentials of Qigong practice.

Fig. 2. Classification of Qigong

- Qigong
  - External
  - Internal
    - Dynamic — Emphasis on physical exercise of body
    - Static
      - Emphasis on breath exercice
      - Emphasis on mental concentration

II Psychology and Behavioral Science of External Qigong

As a branch of Qigong exercise, external Qigong appeared about 16 years ago and became widely accepted. This was at a time when Qigong practice became more and more popular and widely adopted to treat diseases and preserve health among Chinese people. However, as a particular therapy it was named Buqi (distributing Qi) in the ancient medical literature. It means a therapy to deliver the Jingqi (material or energy) from the bodies of the practitioners to patients' bodies for curing their diseases and it is similar to the Mesmer (1734--1815) method and the magnetic theory of animals developed in France in the 18th century. External Qigong is actually a hypnotherapy by suggestion developed from the Yuanqi Lun (theory of primordial Qi) of traditional Chinese medicine from the ancient times of China, i.e. much earlier than the appearance of the magnetic theory of animals.

By the end of the 70s, some physicists, who were deficient in their knowledge of both psychology and hypnotism by suggestion, found signals of micro-particle flow produced by Qigong specialists when they were delivering external Qi. Their further studies proved the presence of signals of static electricity, magnetism, micro-particle flow,

bio-mechanics and sub-audible sound and then they built a hypothesis about the material nature of external Qi. However, this hypothesis has been disproved by the results of more and more new research. Bio-physical phenomena, like the weak sonic, photic, electric and magnetic changes on the body surface of human beings are the natural bio-physical phenomena of animals, although they can be magnified by the Qigong specialists during their practice of Qigong, especially when they concentrate their minds at certain spots or places for a long time (a physiological reaction to psychological activity). However, as proved by much research work, the bio-physical changes are too weak and too limited in area to produce a substantial physiological or therapeutical reaction in the human body. Up to the present time none of them could provide convincing evidence to prove that an apparent physiological change in the receivers of external Qi can be produced by those weak bio-physical changes of Qigong practitioners, although they are positioned very close to each other. What can be produced is only the subjective sensations mentioned by the receivers of external Qi. This is a psychological effect and, to the seemingly scientific hypothesis of the physicists, it is induced by belief in primordial Qi. Therefore, external Qigong is actually a psychological phenomenon and it is an important project of psychological investigation in terms of the regional culture, "scientific" belief system and one's reaction to suggestion [1].
External Qigong is also different from the western hypnotism by suggestion. The psychological effect of the latter is produced by speech, but in traditional external Qigong it is produced by various physical actions and behaviors, accompanied by sound and music, acupuncture and massage management. The receivers of external Qigong think that they may receive some unknown essential materials or primordial Qi, and that they may obtain various subjective sensations produced by unknown materials or primordial Qi. Consequently Chinese patients may enjoy a great mental satisfaction, produced by the oriental pattern of suggestion through physical action, rather than the western pattern of suggestion in speech [2]. The desire of the patients to obtain medical care by means of receiving certain medical materials can be satisfied through the procedure of delivering Qi and receiving Qi. This was a great discovery in China and also a wonderful application of psychology by suggestion among oriental people.

Tab. 1: Comparison between Qigong and hypnotism

	Qigong	Hypnotism
Time of invention	4000 years ago	Late 18th Century
Region of application	China	Western countries
Theoretical basis	Primordial Qi theory	Magnetic theory of animals
Techniques	Psychological suggestion & behavioral adjustment	Psychological suggestion

III Psychology and Behavioral Science of Internal Qigong

The fundamental study of internal Qigong is to investigate the methods and effects of the 3 important essentials of Qigong practice.

1 Mental exercise of Qi-gong

Exercise of the mind is always emphasized as the most important aspect of Qigong practice and it is actually a psychological exercise. Exercise of mind is a kind of psychological exercise done by the practitioners themselves through some psychological activities, such as imagination and concentration of attention. The exercise of mind may be rich and colorful, People may think of the scenery as pleasing to both eye and mind, as delightful natural phenomena or comfortable sensation in their bodies. The exercise of mind in Qigong practice is actually a process to concentrate one's attention, and a means concentrate one's mind. For example, attention may be concentrated at a spot, like Dantian, Baihui (GV 20), etc. Attention may also be slowly and regularly shifted along a course to produce a specific sensation in the body, such as along the small Zhoutian or large Zhoutian meridian. No matter through what kind of psychological activity one performs the exercise of mind, it is always a kind of psychological self-training of mind to improve the function of the brain. Therefore, the exercise of mind in Qigong practice is theoretically the same as that in auto-hypnotism, but the invention and development of Chinese Qigong exercise is always guided by the traditional medical theories, especially by theories of Qi, blood and meridians. Those theories are also used to guide the application of the methods of Qigong exercise by practitioners; to detect a specific sensation in the human body during Qigong practice; and to explain the therapeutic mechanism of Qigong therapy [3]. However, our ancestors could not use psychological and physiological knowledge to explain the Qigong exercise because of historical limitations, although they discovered and developed countless methods of Qigong exercise. As with external Qigong, they used the theory of primordial Qi to explain the mechanism of internal Qigong exercise. This is a theory about the change of materials in the body, and practitioners may feel a satisfaction in obtaining the means and materials for the preservation of their physical and mental health when they are performing the tedious psychological training. This is a reason why the Qigong exercise could survive and develop over thousands years from ancient times, and more and more practitioners would adhere to Qigong exercises year by year.

It should be emphasized that the requirements of body posture, to practice the exercises, must be strictly fulfilled, even when people are performing the still exercise of the mind. In psychological training the posture of the body is not a requirement to be fulfilled. There are 3 postures for the practice of internal Qigong exercise, namely the standing, sitting and lying postures. Although there is no visible movement of the body in the sitting posture, the upper body should be kept erect, the chest drawn in, the back straightened, the shoulders and elbows drooped down, the spine maintained straight and the whole body adequately relaxed. This sitting posture is described as "to sit like a bell" (like a big bronze bell in a temple). it is actually a motionless physical exercise of the body. Besides the maintenance of body posture like a big bell, the mind should also keep thinking of its bell-like body. What is the beneficial psychological and physiological effect of this posture? In the sitting posture the drawn-in chest can support the straightened back and the straightened back may increase the elasticity of the muscles attached to the spinal column. This posture, with shoulders and elbows drooped down, may help the relaxation and elongation of muscles between the shoulder, elbow, wrist and finger joints. The relaxation and elongation of muscles may produce 4 beneficial effects: (1) The number of patent capillary blood vessels in the muscles and the volume and speed of capillary blood flow may be increased: (2) cellular metabolism and all physiological activities may be improved; (3) the exchange of gases in muscles and other tissues may be enhanced; and (4) the supply and consumption of oxygen may be increased [4]. This specific training of internal Qigong is different from that of the auto-hypnotism and psychological training. The persistent practice of the exercise of mind may apply a remarkable beneficial influence to the mental and psychological activities of human beings.

2. Breath exercise of Qigong

Different methods of breathing exercise, such as regular abdominal breathing, reverse abdominal breathing or fetal breathing may be performed to produce a remarkable effect to the human body through the expansion of chest, increase in vital capacity, movement of the diaphragm, peristalsis of the stomach and intestines, and massage of internal organs to adjust the functions of the respiratory, digestive and vegetative nervous systems. Therefore, it is different from that of auto-hypnotism. At the same time, practitioners are asked to concentrate their mind by repeatedly and silently reading a sentence, for example, a particular sentence with 6 Chinese words, so that the cerebral cortex can be maintained in a condition of supression and inhibition. The breathing exercise with silent reading of a sentence contains the conscious or subconscious psychological training of auto-hypnotism, but according to the principles and methods of the breathing exercise, the therapeutic effect of this exercise is obtained mainly through the adjustment of mental and physical activities, which is an internal behavior of the practitioners themselves.

3. Daoyin (dynamic) exercise of Qigong

In western countries the dynamic exercise of Qigong is called Qigong gymnastics, because the exercise of body and limbs is much emphasized in dynamic Qigong. However, the Daoyin exercise is different from pure gymnastics because the chief character of this exercise is the combination of dynamic and static exercises together, by mixing the dynamic exercise into the static exercise. and by mixing the static exercise into the dynamic exercise. The mental exercise in the Daoyin exercise is also varied in method. Besides the simple concentration of attention on a particular spot or substance, such as the Dantian point, a limb or a tree, the mind may also concentrated on an abstract figure, such as "spreading wings of roc", "protruding claws of a blue dragon" or "expanding wings of a crane". In the dynamic exercise of Qigong the breath exercise is often much emphasized, but not as much as in static exercise of Qigong. In auto-hypnotism the

Fig. 3 Effects of autohypnotism

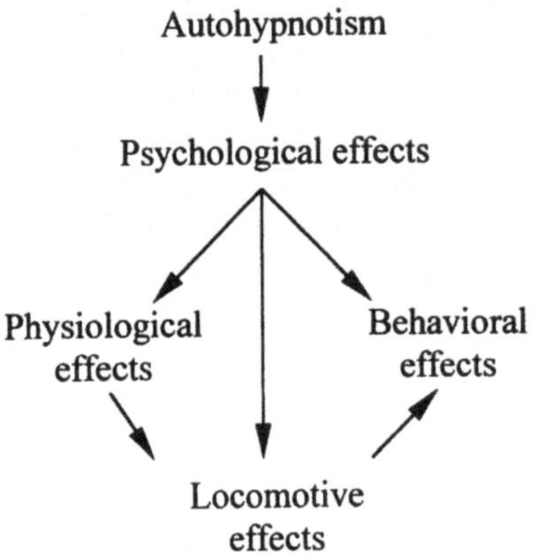

Fig. 4 Effects of internal Qigong

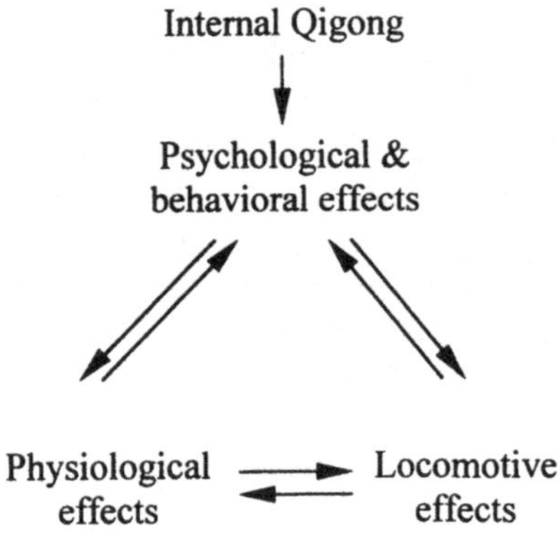

concentration of mind is also much emphasized, but there is not any requirement regarding the movement of limbs or the type of breathing. Although sometimes deep breathing is required in auto-hypnotism, it is only for mental relaxation. In the dynamic exercise the coordinate breathing exercise and the movement of limbs is under the control of a concentrated mind, as psychological training can adjust the mental activities, behaviors and functions of the internal organs. The beneficial effects produced by dynamic Qigong are more remarkable than those produced by auto-hypnotism [3].

The difference of therapeutic effects between auto-hypnotism and internal Qigong exercise can be shown by the following diagrams.

IV Summary

According to the reports of many scientific studies, both external Qigong and hypnotism may produce their effects on the physiological functions and the morphological changes of the human body through psychological adjustments, However, external Qigong is performed by applying the influence of physical actions, and hypnotism is performed by applying the influence of speech. Internal Qigong and auto-hypnotism are all performed through psychological action, but in internal Qigong behavioral training is also emphasized so as to apply its influence on physiological functions and morphological changes of the human body. In both external and internal Qigong psychological and behavioral influences bring about physiological activities and morphological changes. This is just the difference between oriental Qigong therapy and western psychological therapy. Although an important branch of Traditional Chinese medicine, oriental Qigong therapy is not neglectful in its study of psychology and behavioral science.

References

[1] Wang Weidong: (1994): *Various Favorite Problems of Qigong*, published by Publisher of Aviation Industry.

[2] Wang Weidong & HarukiYutaka:(1995): *Analysis of Behavioral Factors in External Qi Therapy of Qigong*, published by Japanese Society of Hypnology.

[3] Wang Weidong:(1990):Qigong exercise and autohypnotism. *Journal of Qigong*.

[4] Xue Ligong & Wang Weidong:(1990): *Chinese Medical Qigong*, published by Heilongjiang Publisher of Sciences and Technology.

"TIBETAN MEDITATION, YOGA AND HEALING PRACTICES: MIND-BODY INTERCONNECTIONS"

Dr. Elisabeth A. Stutchbury,
Australian Research Council, Post Doctoral Fellow, Anthropology,
Australian National University, Canberra, AUSTRALIA

ABSTRACT

Despite considerable fascination with some of the apparently 'magical' aspects of various Tibetan Buddhist meditation techniques, such as increased body temperature produced in the tummo (Tibetan [hereafter Tib.]: *gTum mo*) or 'psychic heat' practice of the Six Yogas of Náropa, a discourse which gives genuine epistemic status to such 'technologies of consciousness' has not been developed in western academic literature. Drawing on anthropological research conducted in a small western Himalayan hermitage, where these advanced and esoteric yogic meditations are mastered in three year solitary retreats, and on personal experience, I develop a framework for understanding these practices, relating the construct of the mind-body complex to the Tibetan conceptualisation of the harmoniously balanced elemental body. Some of the implications for modalities of healing in the western context are then briefly explored.

EMERGENT UNDERSTANDINGS AND THE TECHNOLOGY OF CONSCIOUSNESS

In the past three decades, the western fascination with eastern religions and philosophies that has permeated popular culture has also received considerable attention in some side alleys of mainstream academic research, including numerous studies of the physiological and biological effects of various meditation techniques. Although these investigations have been developed in several disciplines within the academy, it is the popular publications, written for a larger audience, which have garnered greatest attention and also broken disciplinary boundaries. Changes in understandings and connections between disciplines previously separate have resulted in the emergence of new disciplines, notably cognitive sciences. In this domain the interdependence between the functioning of the mind and various physiological processes of the human body are paramount.

Research into the effects of meditation and yoga, and thus the interface between religious or philosophical systems, and science, particularly in the form of 'east meets west' constitutes a significant part of the emergent discourse exploring the convergences between paradigms, which continues to find its greatest expression in publications where the distinction between academic and popular writing is blurred, as evidenced, for instance, by Goleman's recent Emotional Intelligence (1996). This empowers the discourse. However emergent understandings are sometimes slow to filter through to some academic writings, and certainly much of the popular literature remains firmly limited, a point to which I will return later.

This discussion furthers the discourse, laying bare the challenges encountered in exploring understandings derived from different paradigms. I take as a starting point this dialogue between science and Tibetan Buddhism, fostered in recent years by His Holiness the Fourteenth Dalai Lama, and presented to the public in books such as Mind-Science: An East-West Dialogue (Goleman & Thurman, 1991), Gentle Bridges: Conversation with the Dalai Lama on the Sciences of Mind (Haywood & Varela, 1992), and The Embodied Mind: Cognitive Science and Human Experience (Varela, Thompson & Rosch, 1993). In particular, I will focus on one particular technique of Tibetan Buddhist meditation, that of tummo (Tib. gTum mo) or 'psychic heat'. This meditation technique has already received attention in this discourse which has begun the exploration of the convergences between the two paradigms, one Western and the other Tibetan.

To date, the dialogue around tummo has been limited. On the one hand we have an analysis by Herbert Benson, using perspectives derived from scientific research onto the physiological and neuro-physiological effects of the heat generating yoga (Benson, 1991). We also have a very different account from Robert Thurman, presenting the yoga in terms of the Tibetan Buddhist philosophical understanding (Thurman, 1991). Goleman has drawn attention to the challenges raised by this advanced meditative yoga and these two contrasting accounts of it, within the context of the meeting of paradigms, using perspectives derived from psychology and the cognitive sciences (Goleman, 1991).

I intend to broaden the discourse principally through offering an appreciation of this meditation practice as a 'technology of consciousness' which gives genuine epistemic status to Tibetan Buddhist systems of knowledge, particularly the modality of healing. I draw on insights gained through my own involvement with Tibetan meditational practices, and from the anthropological field work I conducted in the western Himalaya, in order to contextualise and articulate my current appreciation of the knowledge and wisdom embedded in Tibetan Buddhist technologies of consciousness, and in particular the heat generating practice of tummo.

Tummo's Fascination and the Western Gaze

Herbert Benson, Tummo and the Lama

Herbert Benson, well known for his pioneering work in Mind/Body research at the Harvard Medical School, began investigating the various physiological and neuro-physiological effects of meditation in 1967, with some subjects who practised Transcendental Meditation. From these early experiments, Benson developed the notion of the 'relaxation response', a technique which elicits the physiological changes understood to be the opposite in effect to the stress or 'fight-or-flight' response. He formulated a simple two step technique and published his first popular self-help book in 1975. Since then, the relaxation response has become the mainstay of self-help techniques offered by Benson and his colleagues in treating a variety of medical complaints, including high blood pressure, asthma, infertility and insomnia, scientifically researched at the Harvard Medical School, the Mind/Body Institute and the Deaconess Hospital. Some of the research findings have been published in appropriate scientific journals (eg. Benson, Malvea & Graham, 1973), as well as presented to a much larger public in popular self-help books on healing, and optimising change and human potential (Benson, 1975; Benson & Proctor, 1985; Benson & Proctor, 1988; Benson & Stark, 1996).

Benson's interest in the physiological changes he has observed in subjects while meditating extends beyond the comparatively simple techniques of Transcendental Meditation. In 1978, not long before his first meeting with H. H. the Dalai Lama, Benson read an account of tummo by Alexandra David-Neel, the French female explorer, who travelled in Tibet in disguise in the 1920's. Tummo has been described by western explorers and Tibetologists, despite the cultural context of this particular meditation practice, which I discuss in more detail later. Tummo is an advanced practice which is transmitted orally and guarded by strict rules and promises made between disciple and teacher. This might be expected to prohibit and limit opportunities for observing the practice. Nevertheless, these early accounts of Tibetan Buddhism, particularly David-Neel's breathtaking adventures and descriptions of extraordinary meditative feats, have been read by many, colouring western perceptions. Furthermore, tummo has become the focus of considerable scientific research, although it is only one of many meditative and yogic practices from the exceedingly rich tradition of Tibetan Buddhism.

Upon meeting with the Dalai Lama, Benson asked if it would be possible to scientifically study yogis engaging in this practice (Benson & Proctor, 1985 & 1988, & Benson, 1991). I quote:

His Holiness replied, 'It will be very difficult to measure these abilities. The people who practice this meditation do so for religious purposes. It must be experienced in order to feel the benefits. You must experience it first.' Then he added, "Still, our culture is undergoing many changes. We have been forced out of our homeland into exile...perhaps there is some worth in allowing this study to be done.' (Benson, 1991, p. x).

Benson later received an invitation from His Holiness to study three practitioners, and in February 1981, the first physiological and neuro-physiological tests of the effects of tummo practice were made in Upper Dharamsala, H. P., India. The results of these tests were published in 1982 in Nature, indicating that the subjects were able to increase the temperature in their fingers and toes by up to 8.3 degrees C or about 15 degrees F. (Benson, et al., 1982a). Two letters questioning the validity of the published findings, and Benson's response, appeared three issues later (Benson, 1982b). I am not in a position to evaluate the scientific validity or otherwise of these tests, and the strength of the criticism levelled against the results. Benson, apparently determined to gain irrefutable evidence, further negotiated with H. H. the Dalai Lama. With permission in hand, Benson went to India with a film crew early in 1985, and in a small gonpa (Tib. dgon pa) literally meaning 'a place of solitude' and frequently glossed as 'monastery', in Manali, filmed several practitioners performing tummo. Unfortunately, we don't have the

footage, so we will make do with the description Benson has made of the event in Your Maximum Mind:
"With a growing sense of excitement, the filmmakers set up their equipment in the small monastery. They waited expectantly in the chilly room until about 3:00 A.M., when twelve monks entered. The indoor temperature was just 40 degrees Fahrenheit. The monks proceeded to take off all their clothes, except for small loincloths. The monks then assumed a cross-legged posture on the floor. They dipped cotton sheets, measuring three feet by six feet, into pails of water that had been placed in front of them; the water was about 49 degrees Fahrenheit.
Under the supervision of the monastic master, they thenicked up the sopping wet sheets, wrung them out to get rid of the excess water, and then wrapped them around their upper bodies. The sheets were so wet that the cloths lay translucent against the monks' bodies: Their skin could be seen clearly through the wetness.
At this point the monks started to practice their *gTum-mo* Yoga meditation - and an amazing phenomenon began to occur. Although most people would have begun to shiver violently when exposed to such cold wetness, these monks didn't react at all. Instead, they sat calmly, and within three to five minutes, the sheets wrapped around them began to *steam*! The room filled with water vapour so that the lenses of the cameras became fogged over and had to be wiped off constantly. Within thirty to forty minutes, the sheets draped around the monks were completely dry.
Then the monks started all over again. They dipped another set of sheets into cold water, wrung them out to some extent and draped these over their shoulders. As before, the monks began practicing their *gTum-mo* meditation. Again the steaming started in three to five minutes, and the sheets were completely dry in another half an hour or so. They then repeated the process once again. Although the entire ceremony took several hours, not once did the monks who were participating shiver or shake from the cold. Nor did they show any other signs of discomfort" (Benson & Proctor, 1988, pp. 18-19).
It is an interesting co-incidence that the practitioners filmed by Benson and his crew are well known to me, although I had left India early in 1984, the year before this film was made. I had conducted my own research at this very same small gonpa in Manali, using rather different methods from those employed by Benson et al. (and although I would very much have liked to use the medium of film, the resources for making an ethnographic film were not available to me at that time). Moreover, I lived in the northwest Himalaya for three and a quarter years, during my initial anthropological fieldwork, returning to visit for five weeks in 1992. This serendipitous co-incidence provides the basis for my contribution to the discourse between the two paradigms, one western and the other Tibetan.

Náropa, Tummo and Drukchen Rinpoche

Although the people with whom I lived are adept at the heat generating practice of tummo, they had impressed the importance of its secret transmission upon me, and with due respect, I explored the lives of these practitioners, and in particular, the relationship between village and gonpa, or place of meditation. I collected details of the practice lineages of the Drukpa Kargyu ('brug pa bka' brgyud Tib.), one of the orders of Tibetan Buddhism to which the people that I lived with belong. Because these yogis are adept at a series of practices called the Six Yogas of Náropa, which includes tummo, I collected a great deal of information about the practice lineage associated with tummo, both the historical and cultural context of the practice, as well as the social context - details about the meditation retreats and life at the gonpa.

I also took teachings and engaged in the practice of meditation. My impetus for doing this was twofold. Firstly, I had suffered a lot of ill health, including a severe illness, at fifteen, with an extreme febrile reaction and consequent near death experience. Since that time, I have been plagued by problems indicative of immune deficiency. I was also involved in a major car accident when I was twenty-one. There was much in my life to be healed, physically, emotionally and spiritually, and I had not found the means to do this in my own culture. So when I decided to conduct anthropological research among Tibetan Buddhists, I was determined that as an adjunct to my anthropological research I would find a personal teacher and persue my own healing as well.

Furthermore, when I began to live at the gonpa, a small hermitage, I found that the practitioners spent much of their time in meditation. In the summer months, they would sit quietly on the flat earthen roofs of their small houses, often without moving for hours, apparently just staring into space, across the valley to the twenty thousand foot snow capped peaks. In order to understand what they were doing, my questioning led me to actually begin to practice meditation. There really was no other choice. As I mentioned above, His Holiness had told Benson that it is necessary to experience meditation, to actually use the techniques, in order to appreciate the benefits. I extend that suggestion. It is necessary to experience and use the techniques in order to understand and explain the process of meditation.

However, when I did my doctoral fieldwork, I did not intend to write about the actual practices, to lay bare the inner workings of the practitioner, particularly those that are governed by a strict code of secrecy. When I met with Drukchen Rinpoche ('brug chen rin po che Tib.), the highest reincarnation within the particular lineage of the Drukpa Kargyu that I had been studying in India, five years after my return to Australia, in January 1989, several discussions encouraged me to expand the focus of my research. Drukchen Rinpoche is a well travelled young man, born in 1963. He is considered to be the reincarnation of the Indian siddha Náropa, and consequently to have a special connection with tummo.

Tummo is the first of a series of highly specialised yogic practices known as the Six Yogas of Náropa. The eleventh century Indian Siddha, Náropa (AD. 1016-1100), who developed these yogas and was responsible for transmitting these tantric teachings to the Tibetans. This oral transmission lineage is said to have continued in an unbroken line to the practitioners with whom I studied.

When I met Drukchen Rinpoche in Australia, he showed me a letter which he had received from the host of an American mid-day television program, inviting him, as the reincarnation of the Indian siddha Náropa, to demonstrate tummo in front of a live studio audience. Tummo on national American television! Drukchen Rinpoche was at a loss as to how to appropriately respond to this request which demonstrated a typical western fascination with the 'magical' side effects of meditative practice, in this case the production of body heat, and a complete lack of comprehension and respect for the wisdom and esoteric nature of these practices. As we talked, he suggested that it would be useful if I could provide information on the cultural context of these yogic practices and develop a frame of understanding which would help westerners to appreciate their real significance within the Tibetan Buddhist tradition. This remains an important agenda in my work, and this discussion is an attempt to fulfil that goal.

My quandary is that there is a central and fundamental difficulty in attempting to communicate the technology of consciousness embedded within advanced systems of meditation, such as the 'inner yoga' practices of Náropa. The pathways of the mind-body complex which are mapped in the methods and language used to describe and explain these practices are not readily translatable. How many of you understand what I might be hinting at by the description 'inner yoga', which I have just applied to these Yogas of Náropa? I have used 'inner yoga' to translate the Tibetan tsa-lung (*rtsa rlung*), which corresponds to the Sanskrit 'n' and 'préna', respectively. These terms taken individually can be translated as 'psychic vein' and 'inner air'. I wonder if this careful rendition of these terms has clarified your understanding?

Attempts to render such terminology into another language result in approximations of conceptual understanding overly determined by frames of understanding from a paradigm which has a spurious relationship to the Tibetan system. Recourse to direct experience of the methods may result in a clearer understanding of the technology of consciousness, yet the problem of appropriate conceptual translation remains. However, it is only through such embodied experience that we can challenge the limitations of our habitual analytical ways of thinking and talking about the technology of consciousness, and the potentialities of human experience developed in very different cultural milieux. I shall now describe these yogic practices and their cultural context.

Meditative Training and the Six Yogas of Náropa

The Six Yogas of Náropa belong to the Chagchen (phyag rgya chen po Tib., or MahÉmudrÉ in Sanskrit [hereafter Skt.]) tradition, that is, they employ one of the two principal methods of meditation employed in Tibetan Buddhism, that of transformation. Moreover, the Six Yogas are regarded as very advanced practices, involving transformation practices at the highest level. The yogi or yogini must have quite a deep and stable realisation of õùnyatÉ (Skt. emptiness), the fundamental insight of Buddhist meditation, before it is possible to effectively work with the visualisations of these 'inner yoga' practices. This realisation is gained through thorough training in retreat, involving mindfulness/awareness Buddhist practices.

Rather than generalising, I will speak very specifically about the training undertaken by the Drukpa Kargyu practitioners taught by Gegan Khyentse Gyatso (dge rgan mkhyen brtse rgya mtsho), my first meditation teacher from Apo Rinpoche Gonpa (a pho rin po che dgon pa) in Manali, H. P. This teacher, now in his eighties, is regarded as one of the great masters of the Six Yogas of Náropa. Three practitioners had completed this retreat two years before I commenced fieldwork, and while I was there, a group of seven received instruction, entering into retreat before I left. Since that time, several groups have undertaken and completed their three year retreats, so that the special retreat houses are in constant use - one group finishes and another group then commences their retreat.

Although there is no fundamental reason for this, there is a gender bias in Tibetan culture which is clearly evident in the teaching and transmission of the Six Yogas, for the majority of practitioners are male. This is certainly the case where I conducted my research. Indeed, there is another transmission lineage, known as the Six Yogas of Niguma, which originated with Náropa's sister or consort. These closely related yogas are also still taught and transmitted, and there are teachings from both lineages for female practitioners.

For those students, whether male or female, studying with Gegan Khyentse, the path of practice begins with the teaching of the fundamental teachings of Tibetan Buddhism, 'The Four Thoughts which Turn The Mind towards the Dharma' (Tib. Lo tog nam zhi, blo ldog rnam bzhi), and instructions for the Tantric Preliminary Practices or ng_ndro (sngon 'gro Tib.). This practice is usually performed in a series of four retreats, each lasting for one to two months, or if there is the possibility, in one continuous retreat of six or seven months. During this time the practitioner is engaged for twelve to fifteen hours a day in the visualisations and mantric recitations and other techniques employed. Such retreats are very intensive and the practitioner 're-programmes' his or her mind-body complex, following the precise instructions of the teacher. Gegan Khyentse often requires his students to undertake four or five such retreats.

As well as that, the disciple receives instructions in the fundamental Buddhist practices of mindfulness/awareness - õamatha (Skt..) or shin _ (zhi gnas Tib.), single pointed concentration or calm abiding, and vipaõyané (Skt.) or lhagtong (lhag mthong Tib.), insight meditation, the union of which is méhamudré, and yidam (yi dam) practice, which involves visualisation and transformation into deities embodying aspects of enlightenment. These practices provide a complete path to realisation or enlightenment. However, some students will continue on the path of the tantric adept.

It is only when the master judges the student to be fully prepared that the oral transmission for the Six Yogas of Náropa is given. Then, before the practitioner enters into the strict Náro Ch_drug (náro'i chos drug), or Six Yogas of Náropa retreat, which lasts for three years, three months and three days, according to the Tibetan lunar calendar, they must develop a reasonable proficiency in and understanding of the practices and what is required of them, as a basis for the intense retreat during which they will perfect these yogic practices.

As mentioned above, a small group of practitioners enters into retreat together, each practicing in their own small room, but meeting together for simple meals, which they prepare for themselves. The practitioners remain in strict isolation from the outside world for the duration of the retreat, although able to confer with their teacher, and perhaps also with one other adept, appointed to guide the retreat, who will visit on a regular basis to ensure that there are no difficulties arising in the practice. During the retreat the practitioners do not cut their hair, symbolising that they have cut their attachments to the outside world. After the retreat, the appearance of the previously shaven-headed practitioners is significantly altered, an outward symbol of the inner changes wrought on their being through this period of intense meditative practice.

The Six Yogas retreat begins in autumn, and involves many hours of meditation each day. Meditation practice develops with such intensity that even when asleep, the practitioner is engaged in the 'dream yoga' and 'clear light' practices. The other four yogas are practised according to season, and so are repeated as the years pass. The first of these yogas is the 'psychic heat' practice, tummo or candálí (Skt.). The practitioner must gain expertise in this practice before he or she can proceed with the other yogas. A brief description of the Six Yogas follows:

1. **Tummo** (*gtum mo,* canálí - Skt.) or 'psychic heat' is developed with trulkor (*'phrul 'khor*) or physical exercises in the autumn, and in winter the tummo continues with rékyang (*ras kyang*) and répu (*ras pu*), in which the body heat generated by the yogi, while meditating out in the snow at night, is used to quickly dry the robes which have been soaked;
2. **Gyulu** (*rgyu lus*), the 'illusory body' practice, is for recognising the illusions of saäsÉra (Skt.) or cyclic existence, and is undertaken in Spring;
3. **Milam** (*rmi lam*), the 'dream yoga' is practised every night while sleeping; as is
4. **Osal** (*'od sal*), the 'clear light' practice;
5. **Bardo** (*bar do*), the 'intermediate state' practice for after death is pursued in early summer; and
6. **P'owa** (*'pho ba*), the 'transference of consciousness' practice, preparation for the time of death, is performed for one week only.

Evaluations: Scientific and Popular

Indeed, tummo, or the psychic heat practice, is fundamental to all highest level tantric teachings, and over the years this yogic feat has gained considerable attention from western observers, as we have seen. Some have made the assumption that the practice of producing body heat, which is demonstrated by the drying of wet robes in the snow during the winter, is necessary for yogis living in the high and cold terrain ofTibet and the Himalaya. Some view the practice as some sort of magical accomplishment or power, like being able to levitate or fly through the air.

Some take the perspective of the sceptic, and view this practice, and all other 'magical' accomplishments as fraudulent hocus pocus. For instance, in 1991 the Newcastle (N.S.W. Australia) branch of the Sceptic Society organised a lecture by Mr. B. Pramanand at the University of Newcastle, where I was teaching at the time. This was reported on the front page of the Newcastle Herald. Mr Pramanand has been given a scholarship by the Government of India in order to train individuals to expose the fraudulent and fake 'god men' of India - the babas and sadhus who pierce their bodies and tongues with hooks and trident ended arrows, playing on people's beliefs and gullibility and extracting rupees from them in the process. Mr Pramanand is reported to have said that: "...as for those that are claimed to endure freezing temperatures in the snow, clad only in a cloth, this is easily achieved by covering the body in yak's butter." (Newcastle Herald).

Benson and his colleagues have provided us with enough scientific data to cast doubt on Pramanand's assertion that those that claim to be able to increase body temperature through specific meditation techniques are really tricksters, who simply insulate themselves against the cold with yak butter. But do the results gained by the technologies of western scientific endeavour tell us anything about the technology of consciousness, the specific techniques and methods which produce these results?

I think not. These appraisals are completely missing the point, or at the very least, they are talking about the phenomena within an alien frame of reference, and without entering into a meaningful dialogue which might really lead to insight into the capabilities and working of the mind-body. In Your Maximum Mind, admittedly a book for popular consumption, Benson suggests that the basis of the heat generating ability of the monks who featured in his film is the 'relaxation response'.

I am certainly not the first to observe that the techniques of the relaxation response correspond very closely to one of the most basic Buddhist meditation techniques of (õamatha (Skt) or shin_ (zhi gnas. Tib.), single pointed concentration, or calm abiding, as well as to basic meditative techniques from several other religious traditions (see eg. Goleman, 1991). As I've mentioned, méhamudré meditation, the union of calm abiding and single pointed meditations are practiced during the Six Yogas retreat. However, this is only one of several meditation techniques used, and reducing the technology of consciousness employed by these practitioners to the 'relaxation response' fails to elucidate the highly specialised and complex processes occurring.

With regard to Buddhist meditation techniques, it is also quite clear that Benson has developed his appreciation of the essential methods and incorporated the techniques of vipaõyané (Skt.) or lhagtong (lhag mthong Tib.), insight meditation, combining the two methods for the activation of the 'Principle of Maximum Mind' (Benson & Proctor, 1988). These techniques, as presented by Benson, do not lead to the insight and wisdom of méhamudré, nor to the accomplishment of tummo.

I continue with a quotation from Benson's Your Maximum Mind:

"Although we don't have all the answers yet, some further explanations have been offered for their powers.

One leading theory is that the monks have engaged in a process called nonshivering thermogenesis. This involves the ability of the body under some circumstances to burn or metabolize a type of fat called brown fat, which is able to generate very large amounts of heat. In the past, scientists thought that only certain types of non-human mammals, especially those which hibernate, could burn this type of fat. But now it appears that human beings may also have the capacity to generate heat from this fat. We have hypothesised that the monks may have learned to do so through the use of generally unknown powers of the mind.

In any case, it's clear that our minds and bodies are capable of feats heretofore believed impossible - including, but certainly not restricted to, overcoming the effects of severe cold" (Benson & Proctor, 1988, pp. 21-22).

While this hypothesis seems to sound more scientifically plausible to the layman, I do not think it is much of an improvement on Pramanand's yak butter idea.

In his latest book Timeless Healing: The Power and Biology of Belief, again a book for popular consumption, after more experiments on yogis in Sikkim in 1988, Benson suggests the ability of these practitioners to be a result of the faith factor, a potential that opens through the use of the relaxation response:

"Indeed, having documented the mind-boggling physical feats that the monks performed by way of the faith factor, I was curious about how far faith might go. With such a strong faith propelling believers, and channelled through proven mental focusing techniques, I wondered if other 'superhuman' stunts were possible. On other expeditions, my colleagues and I tried to confirm legendary reports that Tibetan monks levitate, rising and hovering above the ground in meditation. But when we were allowed to view the levitation of monks in the mountain hamlet of Chail, it appeared only to be an act of considerable physical agility, in which monks, leg-locked in lotus position, sprang several inches off the floor. They did not hover....
I don't believe it is possible to hover or to perform other physical feats that defy Newtonian physics" (Benson & Stark, 1996, p. 166).

Generally speaking, Benson's formulation of meditation for healing and self-help owes much to those Buddhist meditations which fall under the rubric of mindfulness/awareness practices (Varela, Thompson & Rosch, 1993). Indeed, it is reasonable to suggest that the 'relaxation response' is an ecumenical, cross-cultural approach to meditation technique. Although I have no doubt that Benson and his colleagues are presenting techniques in a fairly straightforward manner, and assisting many people in their processes of healing, I feel that such a presentation of this technology of consciousness derived from the Tibetan Buddhist tradition does not do justice nor offer any new insight into the complexity of mind-body interactions. Rather, it is dismissive of any phenomena that do not neatly fit into a very limited analytical frame of understanding.

At the beginning of my presentation, I asserted that much of this dialogue between the two paradigms is occurring in the realm where the distinction between academic and popular writing is blurred, and that, furthermore, although there is a potential for an empowered discourse, emergent understandings are sometimes slow to filter through to some academic writings, and certainly much of the popular literature remains firmly limited. Put simply, then, I find that Benson and his colleagues have not given genuine epistemic status to the technology of consciousness embedded in the mind-body interactions that occur in tummo, and other inner yoga practices.

Emergent Understandings

I have already suggested that it is necessary to actually gain experience in the meditative processes involved in order to really develop a deeper understanding. Furthermore, we are then faced with the difficulty of making appropriate translations as well as developing an expanded vocabulary which can accommodate emergent meanings. The neuro-physiological approach, whilst furthering the dialogue between biomedicine, with its limited scientific analytical framework, and the Tibetan understanding of healing and balance, involving a realised or enlightened state which is embodied through a meditative process, does not bridge the gap. A framework which provides context and understanding of these technologies of consciousness requires much deeper work which integrates direct experience with analysis. I find that those people who are really breaking ground in this area all share a deep involvement with and respect for the techniques and insights offered by the Tibetan wisdom tradition.

As Varela, Thompson and Rosch, conclude in their essay 'What Do We Mean "Human Experience"':
"It is necessary to have a disciplined perspective on human experience that can enlarge the domain of cognitive science to include direct experience. We suggest such a perspective already exists in the form of mindfulness/awareness meditation. Mindfulness/awareness practice, phenomenological philosophy, and science are human activities: each is an expression of our human embodiment. Naturally, Buddhist doctrine, Western phenomenology, and science are each heir to numerous doctrinal disputes and conflicting claims. Each, however, insofar as it is a form of experimentation, is open to everyone and may be examined with the methods of each of the others. Thus, we believe that mindfulness/awareness meditation can provide a natural bridge between cognitive science and human experience. Particularly impressive to us is the convergence that we have discovered among some of the main themes of Buddhist doctrine, phenomenology, and cognitive science - themes concerning the self and the relation between subject and object" (Varela, Thompson & Rosch, 1993, p. 33).

The Experience of the Practitioners

Tests in America

I will now amplify the voice of the practitioners of tummo as a small step towards building this framework, initially through turning to a short auto-biography of a yogi who died about seven or eight years ago and which was published in English just after his death. (Lobsang Tenzin, 1991). When in his fifties, sometime in the 1980's, Lobsang Tenzin flew to America for scientific tests. Although I have not yet found mention of this event made in any of Benson's published findings, I am certain that this yogi is one of the three tested by Benson in Upper Dharamsala in 1981, and that these tests were made by Benson or one of his colleagues at the Mind/Body Institute. Lobsang Tenzin states that he encountered many obstacles and difficulties for his practice in the United States, mentioning that the considerable travel involved very much upset the balance of his body.
"Before reaching America I underwent many difficulties. I had to travel from Dharamsala to Delhi in a bus for twelve hours at night on uneven winding roads. This rough ride shook up my body and made me vomit. Then I had to travel on a plane for several hours. I did not get time to rest well.
Through experience I have found that meditation is very much related to climatic conditions. When I finally arrived in America day and night were completely reversed from what I was used to. I arrived at ten in the morning, rested the next day and the examination started the day after despite my feeling exhausted which is not conducive to good meditation. Before examining my meditation the doctors took some of my blood. For a tantric practitioner, the red and white drops, of which the blood forms the red, are the essential material which provide the energy of the practice and should not be lost. Consequently after my blood had been taken my body felt heavy and lethargic" (Lobsang Tenzin, 1991, p. 110).
Lama Lobsang Tenzin goes on to describe how over a three day period tests were car-

ried out in a laboratory which was purposefully refrigerated. (It was mid-winter in any case). On the second day they tested his brain and on the third they tested his 'winds and heat'. There were extensive tests carried out before he began meditation, which took about an hour, and for these his upper garments were removed, leaving him wearing only a thin vest. Consequently, he became very cold, his body frozen and shivering, so that when he was asked to begin tummo meditation he encountered difficulty. Even the cushion with which he was provided was discarded, as it was not firm, thus not providing a stable base for his meditation posture. So the Lama sat on the floor. He practised for about a four hour period, changing and modifying the techniques he used to counteract the difficult conditions of the laboratory. During this time the scientists conducted whatever tests they liked. I continue with another quotation:

"Because of the opposing conditions I have mentioned, my meditation was not as strong as usual. [This man had reprogrammed his mind/body to the extent that under normal circumstances he automatically began a light tummo whenever he sat cross-legged] But the scientists who witnessed it thought that it was really marvellous....

When the meditation session was over, I could tell from the scientists' faces that they were satisfied, and they said so too.

With their instruments the scientists could see such things as heat, movement of wind and blood, and my brain waves. There are certain things, however, which cannot be seen by their instruments, such as the non-dual wisdom of great bliss and emptiness, which is the root of all realisation" (Lobsang Tenzin, 1991, p. 111).

Indeed. I doubt that the scientists were able to measure the 'movement of wind and blood', according to the yogi's meaning, whatever else they may have been able to examine. I do not think that the scientists really know of what the yogi is speaking, or where to look, or how to measure. Of course, I would be delighted to see published data on this experiment, which broke through these limitations.

Tests in Manali

I would also very much like to know the results of the tests that were carried out by Benson or his colleagues on three yogis who are well known to me. For the team from Harvard Medical School visited Manali while I was there, and because H. H. the Dalai Lama had requested their collaboration, Gegan Khyentse Gyatso, my teacher and a master of the Six Yogas, Lama Paljor Lharje, a middle aged adept who often assists Gegan when he is teaching, and Lama Kunzang Dorje, who normally resides in one of the caves at Tso Pema (Rewalsar), underwent various tests at the Government Guest House. I have spoken with Lama Paljor about this time on a few occasions. Despite His Holiness' instructions and request, Gegan Khyentse was reluctant to discuss the finer details of the meditation techniques employed, as his commitment to his teaching to orally transmit these teachings only to those who are prepared for them and willing to enter into the transmission, is taken very seriously. Nevertheless, the three yogis were willing to discuss, through a translator, as much as they could to satisfy the enquiries made by the scientist, and certainly obliged with practice for the tests.

When I visited in 1992, I again discussed this occasion, and also the filming of the répu, with Lama Paljor, who found the scientific tests and the filming very strange, and also could not appreciate why the scientists seemed to be so interested in the outward signs, yet didn't really want to know or understand the practices. Certainly, they had no interest in undergoing the rigorous training and retreat necessary to experience the practice.

The limited scientific biomedical framework employed for the tests does not allow an appreciation of realisation or enlightenment as an embodied state, that is, not only as a state which can be measured in various ways (brainwaves, temperature, metabolism and so on), but as a direct, lived, experience, which is not abstracted and disembodied. Another way of framing this is to say that the objective perspective is divorced from the subjective perspective.

Inner Yoga and Embodied States

So, how can we push this analysis and integrate the two paradigms? Is it possible to bridge the gap and come to some understanding of this and other inner yoga practices, and what I have called embodied states?

There is something very specific taking place internally, within the mind/body of the practitioner. It must be clearly understood that the heat that is produced in the body is a by-product or a symptom of specific changes taking place within the mind-body complex of the practitioner, but it is not the aim of the practice. This symptom can be measured with a thermometer. It can be demonstrated just as well through the performance of the répu, the test that is used by the practitioners themselves to display accomplishment and mastery of the inner yoga. When the practitioner is able to quickly dry his (or her) robes with body heat generated through the practice of tummo, at night in the snow in the middle of winter, both the student and the master are certain that the practitioner has accomplished the inner yoga practice and is able to control the movement of energy within the body and so is ready to further develop his or her meditative skills, the sole aim of which is to achieve realisation, or enlightenment. But what is going on, and where, internally?

The subtle energy body and its constituents do not correspond to anything within the biomedical somatic theory and its solid, material, physiological constituents, but seem to arise as a consequence of a technology of consciousness which operates within a mind-body complex. Significantly, different systems of advanced inner yoga meditation manufacture and employ different structures, suggesting that the potentiality for creating these pathways exist, while the actual number of these and the precise location are not fixed in a concrete way. For instance the Hindu system operates a six (or seven) chakra system, while the Tibetan Buddhist system discussed here employs five chakra, and in some Tibetan Buddhist systems only four are used. The most commonly used are the three of the forehead, throat and heart - which within the Tibetan framework correspond to Body, Speech (or the vibrational energy of sound), and Mind respectively.

Through the process of visualisation, energy pathways, or tsa (*rtsa,* nàdí [Skt.]), psychic veins, are created within the body, and then energy, or lung (*rlung*, pràna [Skt.]), is consciously and deliberately moved and manipulated through these pathways, to create the

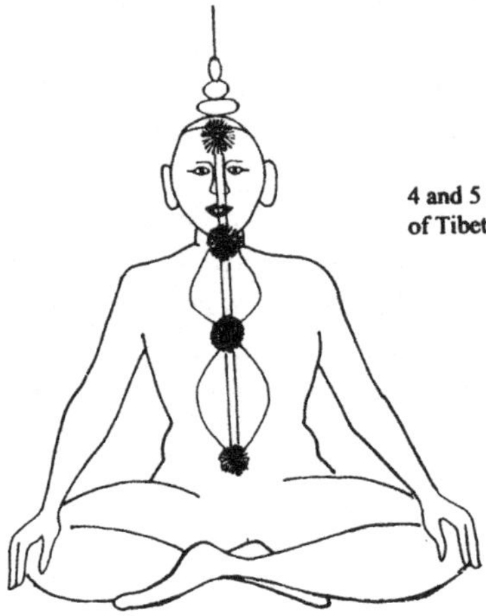

4 and 5 chakra systems of Tibetan Buddhism.

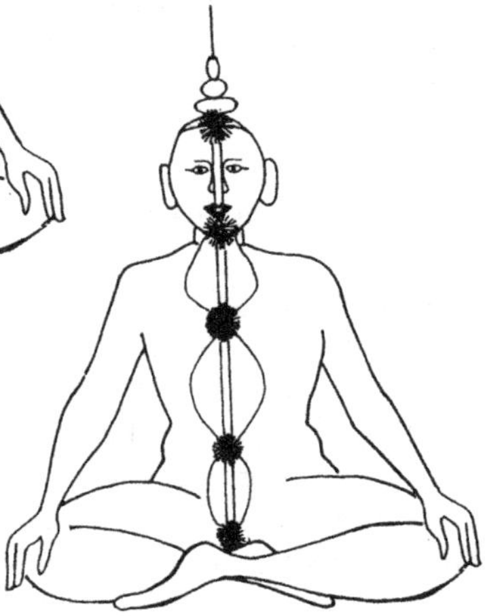

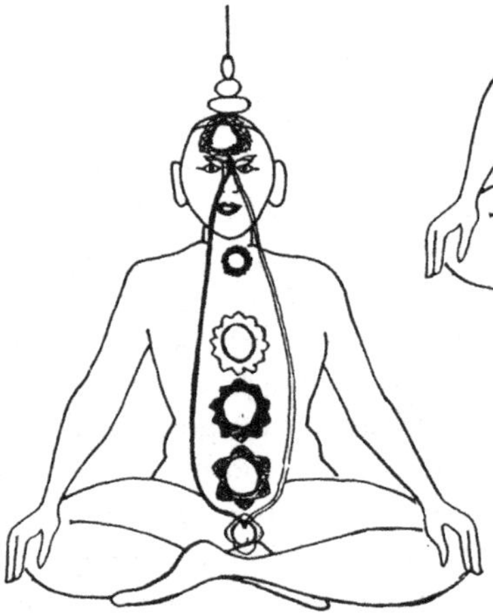

6 chakra Hindu system.

so-called subtle or arcane body, consisting of 'channels' and 'chakras'. The Tibetan term for this subtle body is the 'Illusory Body' (gyulu, *rgyu lus*) which is developed after tummo in the Six Yogas. The subtle body's primary constituents are the central channel, tsa uma (*rtsa dbu ma*, avadhuti [Skt.]), and the right and left channels, tsa roma (*rtsa ro ma*, rásana [Skt.]) and tsa kyangma (*rtsa rkyang ma*, lálana [Skt.]). At several points these channels knot together, creating the chakra (Skt.) or tsa khor (*rtsa 'khor, rtsa yi 'khor lo*), which we can translate as energy centre or channel wheel.

Put very simply, the left and right channels are understood to be polarities: male and female; white and red; skilful means and compassion; attachment or desire and aversion or aggression - these two being the main energies with which we interact with our total environment, and so on. Through the process of visualisation these two main energies are controlled, and at one of the chakra, usually at the navel or the heart, caused to enter the central channel. This mixing of the polar energies causes heat to be generated. The mixed energy is controlled and moved successively through the visualised chakra, which dissolve, open, or unknot, and as this is accomplished the clear light, or osal (*'od sal*), the fourth of the Six Yogas, arises. Put another way, this movement and increase of energy in the central channel causes a transformation of energy, from impure to pure, a kind of 'melt-down' or alchemical process, which creates not only heat within the body, but the illumination of inner light. In this way, the delusion of ignorance or unknowing is purified and in its place arises awareness. According to these conceptualisations, contained in the Tantras, this inner clear light is the ultimate nature of mind, which is pristine, pure, limpid.

For most people, this clear light is experienced but very briefly at the time of death, indeed so briefly that it is not recognised. However, yogis who have developed this inner yoga technique, or others from the repertoire of the higher yogas which have the same result, are able to recognise and to remain in this state after the time of death. Preparation for this occurs during the bardo (*bar do*) the intermediate state practice, which is the fifth of the Six Yogas.

Essentially, in the three year retreat of the Six Yogas, the practitioner learns how to change the inner and outer confusion of existence so that he or she embodies and manifests wisdom, a process which naturally involves healing, at all levels. The practitioner learns how to live well, and to die well. Advanced meditators are able to recognise signs which indicate their approaching death. At the time of death, the accomplished practitioner engages in these inner yoga practices, and the energy contracts to the heart centre. For several days after death the body retains its elasticity, and warmth can be felt above the heart centre. In October 1981, H. H. Sixteenth Gyalwa Karmapa died in the American International Clinic in Zion, near Chicago, Illinios, after a long experience of cancer. Thus we have this well documented account of such death practices, including the testimony of the physicians who were treating him. I have several other accounts of death practice from my own research, and there are several published accounts, although scientific tests, per se, which might try to establish what indeed is happening at a neuro-physiological level, would be extremely difficult to carry out, if not impossible. H. H. Dalai Lama and Benson have discussed this possibility, with Benson claiming that the difficulty is getting to the scene of death on time (1991, p. 34). I think that what is more at issue is the intrusive nature of the hardware and technology used for these tests, which are likely to interrupt the very subtle nature of the movement and contraction of energy which is taking place.

Microcosm - Macrocosm

There are, however, other conceptual frameworks which we can draw upon to deepen our understanding of what is occurring in these inner yoga practices so that we can have some idea of what is meant when the texts say that the clear light arises. In discussing the processes of tantric transformation, such as those involved in these inner yoga practices, I find it useful to employ the model of microcosm and macrocosm, and the correspondences between them. The process which takes place within the practitioner's body, the microcosm, has effect upon and is reflected in the external environment, the macrocosm. Furthermore, as reported by Lobsang Tenzin in the quotation which I read earlier, "...meditation is very much related to climatic conditions' (Lobsang Tenzin, 1991, p. 110). How? You will remember that Lama Lobsang Tenzin was pointing out that he experienced difficulties with his tummo practice because of his adverse surroundings. But there is more to this correspondence between microcosm and macrocosm.

Several people told me about the miraculous events witnessed two years before I began my fieldwork, which was attributed to the level of accomplishment achieved by the three young men who were engaged in the Six Yogas of Naropa retreat. In the final months, the yogis performed r_pu, through which they demonstrate their ability with the tummo practice, repeatedly drying their wet robes in the snow during the long night. As the sun rose, after the yogis had returned to their retreat house, it was surrounded by rainbows, and snowflakes in the shape of flowers fell from a cloudless sky. There are many other such accounts of dramatic and unusual atmospheric phenomena, both from my own research data, and recorded elsewhere.

Such atmospheric phenomena may be explained in terms of the correspondence between microcosm and macrocosm, which within the discipline of anthropology is considered to be symbolic. That is, it is abstracted and so not considered to be real. Rather, it is understood to be a construction within a particular cultural framework. The people with whom I lived perceived the relationship between microcosm and macrocosm as real, and explained to me that the techniques of the inner yoga, which occurred within the microcosm of the yogis' mind-body complexes, were mirrored in the macrocosm, the surrounding environment. Within the Tibetan tradition, unusual atmospheric phenomena are regarded as auspicious coincidences, signs of spiritual realisation, and are frequently reported during the cremation of accomplished practitioners. Again, the cremation of H. H. Sixteenth Gyalwa Karmapa was well documented on film and in several eyewitness accounts.

It is possible to dismiss such occurrences and atmospheric phenomena as either unusual coincidences, mere fantasy, perceptive errors, or fraudulent claims, and engage in a debate which either refutes or accepts such occurrences. Again, however, this is focussing attention on the unusual phenomena, which are symptomatic, a by-product, rather than looking to the underlying principles and the paradigm, which provide a genuine epistemic status for such phenomena.

In the Tibetan tradition, with its refinement of understanding of mind and its nature, the relationship between body and mind, and the way in which experience is embodied, there is, I believe, a powerful framework through which such 'symbolic' correspondence between inner environment (microcosm) and outer environment (macrocosm) can be understood. Moreover, if we can penetrate into the meaning that pertains within this paradigm, we may also find that such correspondences and interdependences actually occur.

It is presumptuous of me to attempt to elucidate the conceptual frameworks which allow this, for it requires drawing upon diverse realms of knowledge and understanding not only from the Tibetan tradition but also including cognitive science, neuro-science, and physics, not to mention meteorology. However, before pointing to key components from the Tibetan cultural arena which, when considered in conjunction with the things I've already discussed, may spark some process which deepens your understanding, I remind you of a quotation I cited earlier, from Varela and colleagues:

"Thus, we believe that mindfulness/awareness meditation can provide a natural bridge between cognitive science and human experience. Particularly impressive to us is the convergence that we have discovered among some of the main themes of Buddhist doctrine, phenomenology, and cognitive science - themes concerning the self and the relation between subject and object" (Varela, Thompson & Rosch, 1993, p. 33).

What we see happening between microcosm and macrocosm hinges on the relationship between subject and object. The relationship between inner yoga practices and the arising of the clear light and auspicious coincidence of atmospheric phenomena presents an area of convergence. The serious exploration of such phenomena, from whatever perspectives that can be brought to bear, is likely to provide insights and shifts in understanding.

Locating the Mind

The Tibetan term sem (sems) has been variously translated as 'mind', or 'spirit' and 'spirituality'.0 These terms have meaning which is not appropriate to the Tibetan conception, nor do they convey what sem is. Sem rides on the energy which moves through the psychic veins, and thus is involved in the visualisations which are made in the inner yoga practices I have been talking about. In general, Tibetans might indicate that sem is at the heart centre, rather than in the head, which is where we are most likely to locate our 'mind'. Perhaps the most useful term I have heard used to translate sem is heart/mind, as it indicates the connections through the energy pathways of the central channel and the movement of sem along those pathways.

Indeed, establishing and working with these connections, so that we are no longer faced with the duality of the rational mind and the emotional heart, for instance, is really the basis of all meditation and spiritual practice. To put it another way, within the integrated mind/body, we can overcome our habitual ways of dealing with our experiences, with what we experience in our outer environment, as either something we desire and grasp, or something that annoys us and we therefore reject. Not only does this conflict or duality dissolve, but through this embodied experience which occurs at very subtle levels of consciousness, and which gives rise to the realisation of the nature of mind, the clear light, the outer environment is affected, as a symptom or by product, so to speak. Again, I am pointing to the relationship between subject and object, and more particularly, to our subjective experience and the objective outer world.

The Elements

As presented in the Tibetan Tantras, the cause through which this correspondence works and has effect is that all matter is constituted of the elements - space, wind or air, water, fire and earth. The effect of the inner yoga practices on the elements which constitute the yogi's body find particular correspondence within the outer elements of the environment. A complete presentation of this material is complex, for it encompasses the theoretical base of the Tibetan medical system.

Moreover, the discourse occurring between paradigms, the east meets west dialogue in physics, particularly quantum mechanics, suggests a fruitful avenue of elucidation for the analysis of the processes that are detailed in the Tibetan conceptualisations. Whilst a presentation of the relevant material is well beyond the scope of my expertise and this paper, it is important to appreciate that the understanding embedded within the Tibetan technology of consciousness, and fundamental to the modality of healing, is that the gross material elements, when purified, dissolve and become light. Each element corresponds to a particular colour: space is blue; wind or air, green; water is white; fire, red; and earth yellow. The death process is understood as the dissolution of the elements, associated with the diminishing of the perceptive capacity of the sense organs, one by one. The dissolution of the death process is the reverse of aggregation which occurs at the time of conception (Namkhai Norbu, 1983).

This understanding is fundamental to the instructions for the dying that are contained in the famous teachings of the Bardo Th_dr_l (bar do'i thos grol), so called The Tibetan Book of the Dead, which is better translated as The Great Liberation Through Hearing in the Bardo. Of course, I am not about to present these teachings, but I wish to very simply present the theoretical framework which underpins both the death process and the practices of inner yoga.

As each element dissolves, a light of that colour arises in the inner perception of the dying person. In the death process, when all the elements have dissolved, i.e. when all the colours of the spectrum are present, the white clear light of the moment of death arises. For most people death comes quite quickly, and because of fear or other emotional confusion surrounding death, these arisings and the clear light are not recognised. However, for the practitioner accomplished in the Six Yogas (or other inner yoga practices), because of their familiarity with the arising of the clear light, they enter into the meditation of that state and remain in it. Thus, for perhaps two or three days, and for as long as a week, the body of the practitioner remains elastic and supple and the heart centre warm, until their meditation in the clear light is finished. Given this elemental composition of the body, and the way in which the inner yoga practices purify through transformation, thus giving rise to the clear light, it is clear why the inner yoga practices also profoundly effect the health and well being of the practitioner.

In Buddhist philosophical terminology, our normal perception pertains to the level of the Nirmànakàya (Skt.) or the 'emanation body'. The level of energy, the 'symbolic' level, is the Sambhogakàya (Skt.), a more subtle manifestation; and the Dharmakàya (Skt.) is the level of the nature of mind. At this point, I would like to suggest that in western theoretical terms, that which is considered to be 'symbolic' may well be found to pertain to a level of perception associated with energy and its manifestation which is coexistent with, yet beyond, our normal perception of the material world.

The Six Yogas and other practices like them work with the Sambhogakàya level, using relative methods to find the absolute. The methods of transformation and visualisation use the mind's ability to construct and manipulate in order to ultimately exhaust that process and bring realisation. This process or technology of consciousness turns the mind inward on the mind-body complex in order to construct and find something, but this is grounded in the realisation of õùnyaté, as I've already mentioned. From this the yogi or yogini realises how the mind works which leads to the absolute realisation of the nature of mind.

Convergences and Pushing the Dialogue

Two Hemispheres - Four quadrants

Research into brain functions and the cognitive sciences is growing rapidly, and I do not pretend to be an expert in this arena. Recently, however, I have had the opportunity to discuss these areas of research with Professor Richard Silberstein, from the Neuro-Science Department at Swinburne University, in Melbourne, Australia. His research focuses on the intersection of brain sciences and physical sciences, particularly explor-

2 HEMISPHERS - 4 QUADRANTS

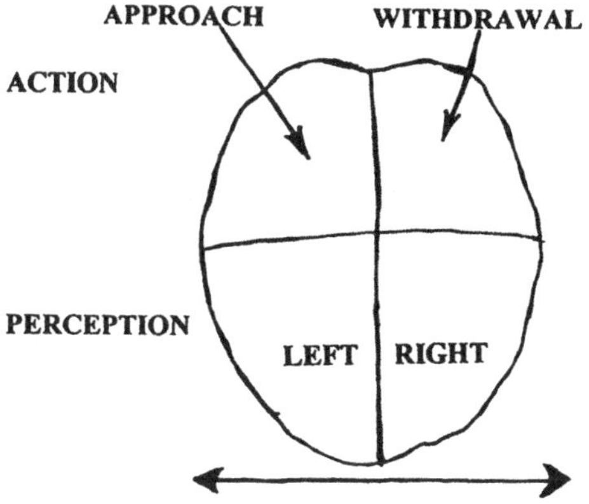

VISUALISATION

INNER YOGA

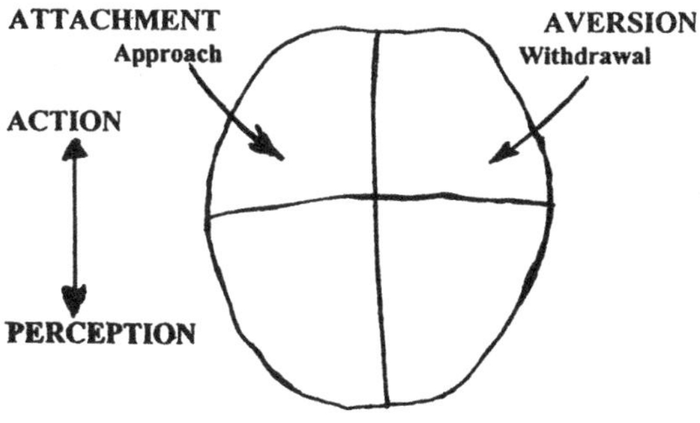

ing technologies which can examine brain activity associated with cognition. He presented a four quadrant model to me which refines the Left/Right brain functions which are now already familiar to us. By introducing the refinements of 'action' and 'perception' to the front and back sections of the brain, as Silberstein suggests, we can see that the process of visualisation in the inner yoga practices, is mapped in a way which allows for integration of left and right hemispheres and perceptual changes which are part of the embodied experience arising out of the use of these technologies of consciousness.

Benson's formulation of Maximum Mind Potential relies very heavily on the left/right hemisphere differentiation. The aim of the game is to allow the right hemisphere to override or short circuit the left. Although he nowhere states this, it is reasonable to assume that his experiments on the yogis practicing tummo revealed marked changes in left/right brain activity, which provided Benson with a clue to developing the Maximum Mind potential framework. Even if inconclusive, it would be very helpful to have access to the full range of neuro-physiological findings of Benson's research, for although the framework is limited, the dialogue and potential for deepening our understanding, particularly where there is convergence between analytical frameworks, is great.

There are many insights which can develop from pushing the dialogue, as His Holiness says:

"(There is a) clear indication of a close link between mind and body: they can be complementary. In light of this, I am very glad to see that some scientists are undertaking significant research in the mind/body relationship and its implications for our understanding of the nature of mental and physical well-being. My old friend Dr. Benson, for example. has been carrying out experiments of Tibetan Buddhist meditators for some years now. Similar research is being undertaken in Czechoslovakia. Judging by our findings so far, I feel confidant that there is still a great deal to be done in the future" (Dalai Lama, 1991, p. 18).

The Immune System

His Holiness also suggest that the specific energy centres in the body, that is the chakra and psychic veins of the subtle body, may "have some connection with what some neurobiologists call the second brain, the immune system. These energy centers play a crucial role in increasing or decreasing the various emotional states within our mind." (Dalai Lama, 1991, p. 18) I find this suggestion very exciting, particularly in the light of my long history of immuno-deficiency, and my process of healing. Although since the advent of AIDS, immune research has increased dramatically, there is still much which is not understood.

We are all aware of the most basic symptom of a healthy immune response to disease - we get a fever. This is a sure sign that our body's immune system is functioning well (Berkow, Fletcher, et al [eds.], 1992; Chrousos, 1995). Now, as we have seen, a rise in body temperature is also a sure sign that the psychic veins and inner airs of the body are being manipulated in a particular way, using a technology of consciousness known as tummo, which when developed gives rise to a state known as clear light, the embodied experience of the state of enlightenment, or realisation - the goal of the path of Buddhist practice. Research into this convergence, through every avenue and discipline possible, will, I think, bear valuable and ground breaking results.

Jonathan Piel (from the Board of Directors) introduces a recent re-publication of a Special Issue of Scientific American entitled Life, Death and the Immune System with these words:

"Ask someone what aspect of his of her being is most essential to that person's unique identity and the reply is likely to be: my mind, or my consciousness. Perhaps, but the immune system might turn out to be a stronger candidate" (Scientific American: A Special Issue, 1994, p. v).

What I am suggesting is that the immune system may turn out to be an aspect of integrated mind/body complex which is not different from the way in which our consciousness, our subtle or higher consciousness, operates within our body - a manifestation of the embodied mind, if you like. While I cannot pretend to be able to substantiate this insight with so called hard scientific evidence, my research, explorations, and personal experience of the technologies of consciousness derived from Tibetan Buddhism, and the Tibetan modality of healing - in short my complete embodied experience, leads me to this conclusion.

Concluding Remarks

I should make it clear that I am somewhat heartened by a scientifically trained doctor of biomedicine who advocates that the mind and body work together, and who encourages patients to meditate, following some sort of guide - albeit their physician who is now also their maximum mind guide. However, after reading several of Benson's popular works, including his latest Timeless Healing: The Power and Biology of Belief (Benson & Stark, 1996), it is not only clear to me that Benson has borrowed much from the Tibetan Buddhist tradition, but also that there is much that he has not really penetrated, or understood.

With a very different agenda, or karmic propensity, my own research of similar meditation techniques led me to a very different involvement. Although my own healing has taken several years, and the process continues, my experiences have convinced me of the power and effectiveness of the spiritual practices of the wisdom teachings of Tibetan Buddhism. From this, enormous respect and devotion has arisen which has continued to motivate my life and academic work. Perhaps one of the most important insights that I experienced directly, and that I grapple with theoretically in my work, is that the mind and body are not separate entities, but are interdependent, although in biomedicine they are usually thought about dualistically. Their relationship is integrated, and healing occurs between the mind and body, bringing physical, spiritual, emotional and mental well-being, which are symptoms of the balance and integration within the mind-body. The understanding resulting from this process within my own life provides the basis for my presentation of working with the mind-body complex.

There are many pieces to the jigsaw which I could choose to expand upon, including details of several different healing meditation practices and my understanding and experience of their effect and relationship with immunity and healing, for instance, for what I am suggesting opens a fascinating dialogue. This, however, awaits another occasion.

There are similarities between the Tibetan Buddhist conceptualisation of the mind-body complex and the constituents of the subtle body with the Chinese concepts of qi and qigong. Anyone familiar with the techniques of acupuncture will have had to grapple with this conceptualisation of body energy and 'meridians', and a way of perceiving the mind and body as a complex which directly challenges western concepts based in the bio-medical dichotomy between mind and body.

The concepts associated with the technology of consciousness in non-western societies have been discussed by anthropologists, and others, but rarely have they been given genuine epistemic status. Western academics engaged in research with Tibetan Buddhism have long been fascinated by the esoteric, but rarely has conceptual knowledge been linked with direct experience of the techniques and methods involved. I suggest that it is only when the two are linked, each informing the other, that it is possible to develop the appropriate concepts to translate the Tibetan Buddhist technology of consciousness.

REFERENCES

Benson, Herbert, Malvea B. P. & Graham J. R. (1973), 'Physiologic Correlates of Meditation and Their Clinical Effects in Headache: An Ongoing Investigation', *Headache,* Vol. 13, pp. 23-24.

Benson, Herbert, (1975), *The Relaxation Response.* New York, William Morrow.

Benson, Herbert, Lehmann J. W., Malhotra M. S., Goldman R. F., Hopkins P. J., & Epstein M. D. (1982a), 'Body temperature changes during the practice of gtum-mo yoga', *Nature,* Vol. 295, pp. 234-236.

Benson, Herbert, (1982b) 'Body temperature changes during the practice of gtum-mo yoga', *Nature,* Vol. 298, p. 402.

Benson, Herbert & Proctor, William, (1985), *Beyond The Relaxation Response.* London, Fount.

Benson, Herbert & Proctor, William, (1988), *Your Maximum Mind.* U.K., Aquarian Press.

Benson, Herbert, Malhotra, M. S., Goldman, R. F., Jacobs, G. D. & Hopkins, P. J., (1990), 'Three case reports of the Metabolic and Electroencephalographic Changes During Advanced Buddhist Meditation Techniques', *Behavioral Medicine,* Vol. 16, pp. 90-95.

Benson, Herbert, (1991), 'Mind/Body Interactions Including Tibetan Studies', in Goleman & Thurman [eds.], pp. 39-48.

Benson, Herbert & Stark, Marg, (1996), *Timeless Healing: The Power and Biology of Belief.* N.Y., Hodder & Stoughton.

Berkow, Robert & Fletcher, Andrew J. et al. [eds.], (1992), *The Merck Manual.* Sixteenth Edition, Rahway, N.J. Merck Research Laboratories. pp. 8-11.

Beyer, Stephan, (1978), *The Cult of Tara. Magic and Ritual in Tibet.* Berkeley, University of California Press. 1st paperback edn.

Blows, Mark, (1992), 'Lifting The Mask: Ways of Working Towards Inner Freedom', *Japanese Journal of Health Psychology,* Vol. 1, No. 1, pp. 90-96.

Capra, Fritjof, (1976), *The Tao of Physics.* Oxford, Fontana.

Capra, Fritjof, (1983), *The Turning Point: Science, Society and the Rising Culture.* London, Flamingo.

Chang, Garma C. C., (1977), *Teachings of Tibetan Yoga*. Secaucus N.J., The Citadel Press.
Chrousos, George P., (1995), 'The Hypothalmic-Pituitary-Adrenal Axis and Immune -Mediated Inflammation', *New England Journal of Medicine*. pp. 1351-1362.
Cozort, Daniel, (1986), *Highest Yoga Tantra. An Introduction to the Esoteric Buddhism of Tibet*. Ithaca, Snow Lion.
Dalai Lama, H. H. Tenzin Gyatso, (1991), 'The Buddhist Concept of Mind', in Goleman & Thurman [eds.], pp. 13-18.
Dalai Lama, H. H. Tenzin Gyatso, (1980), *Universal Responsibility and the Good Heart*. Dharamsala, Library of Tibetan Works and Archives.
Dalai Lama, H. H. Tenzin Gyatso, (1984), *A Human Approach to World Peace*. London, Wisdom Publications.
David-Neel, Alexandra, (1971), *Magic and Mystery in Tibet*. London, Corgi.
Evans-Wentz, W.Y., (1967), *Tibetan Yoga and Secret Doctrines*. 2nd edn. London, Oxford University Press.
Evans-Wentz, W.Y., (1974), *The Tibetan Book of the Dead*. New York, Oxford University Press.
Freemantle, Francesca & Trungpa, Chogyam, (1975), *The Tibetan Book of the Dead, The Great Liberation Throı ?h Hearing in the Bardo*. Boulder & London, Shambhala.
Goleman, Damel and Thurman, Robert A. F. [eds.], (1991), *MindScience: An East - West Dialogue*. The Dalai Lama, Herbert Benson, Robert A. F. Thurman, Daniel Goleman, Howard E Gardner *et alii*. Proceedings of a Symposium sponsored by the Mind/Body Medical Institute of Harvard Medical School & New England Deaconess Hospital and Tibet House New York. Wisdom Publications, Boston.
Goleman, Daniel, (1991), 'Tibetan and Western Models of Mental Health' in Goleman & Thurman [eds.], pp. 90 - 102.
Goleman, Daniel, (1996), *Emotional Intelligence: Why It Can Matter More Than I. Q.* London, Bloomsbury.
Guenther, Herbert V., (1963), *The Life and Teaching of Naropa*. Oxford, Clarendon Press.
Hanson, Judith, (1977), *The Torch of Certainty by Jamgon Kongtrul*. Boulder, Shambhala.
Hayward, Jeremy W., (1987), *Shifting Worlds Changing Minds: Where the Sciences and Buddhism Meet*. Boston & London, New Science Library/Shambhala.
Hayward, Jeremy W. & Varela, Francesco [eds.], (1992), *Gentle Bridges: Conversation with the Dalai Lama on the Sciences of Mind*. Boston & London, Shambhala.
Kalu Rinpoche, (1986), *The Dharma: That Illuminates All Beings Impartially Like the Light of the Sun and the Moon*. Albany, State University of New York Press.
Kelsang Gyatso, (1982), *The Clear Light of Bliss: Mahamudra in Vajrayana Buddhism*. London, Wisdom
Khangkar, Lobsang Dolma, (1986), *Lectures on Tibetan Medicine*. Compiled and edited by K. Dhondup. Dharamsala, Library of Tibetan Works and Archives.
Lauf, Detlef Ingo, (1989), *Secret Doctrines of the Tibetan Books of the Dead*. Boston & Shaftsbury, Shambhala.
Lobsang Tenzin, (1991), 'Biography of a Contemporary Yogi', *Chö-Yang: The Voice Of Tibetan Religion and Culture*, Vol. 3, pp. 102-111.
Mullin, Glenn H., (1985), *Selected Works of the Dalai Lama II*. Ithaca, Snow Lion.
Muses, Charles Arthur, (1961), *Esoteric Teachings of the Tibetan Tantra*. Lausanne, Aurura Press.
Nalanda Foundation, (1985), *The Lion's Roar.* (Video) Narrated by James Coburn. Centre Productions & Shambhala Productions.
Namkhai Norbu, (1983), *On Birth and Life: A Treatise on Tibetan Medicine*. Italy, Shang Shung Edizioni.
Namkhai Norbu, (1986), *The Crystal and the Way of Light: Sutra, Tantra and Dzogchen*. Compiled

and edited by John Shane. New York and London, Routledge and Kegan Paul.

Newcastle Herald, Thursday September 19th, 1991, p.1. Report on B. Pramanand.

Said, Edward W., (1979), *Orientalism.* N.Y., Pantheon Books.

Samuel, Geoffrey B., (1989), 'The body in Buddhist and Hindu Tantra', *Religion,* Vol. 19, pp. 97-210.

Samuel, Geoffrey B., (1990), *Mind, Body and Culture: Anthropology and the Biological Interface.* Cambridge, Cambridge University Press.

Samuel, Geoffrey B., (1993), *Civilized Shamans: Buddhism in Tibetan Societies.* Washington, D. C., Smithsonian Institution Press.

Scientific American: A Special Issue, (1994), *Life, Death and the Immune System.* New York, W. H. Freeman & Co.

Sogyal Rinpoche, (1989), *Dzogchen and Padmasambhava..* Berkeley, Rigpa Publications.

Sogyal Rinpoche, (1992), *The Tibetan Book of Living and Dying.* Edited by Patrick Gaffney & Andrew Harvey, U. K. Random.

Stutchbury, Elisabeth, (1991 unpub.), *Rediscovering Western Tibet: Gonpa, Chorten and the Continuity of Practice With a Buddhist Community in the Indian Himalaya.* PhD dissertation, R.S.Pac.S. ANU.

Stutchbury, Elisabeth, (1991 ms.), 'Tibetan Buddhist Spiritual Practice and Healing Systems.'

Stutchbury, Elisabeth, (1993), 'Working With the Mind-Body Connection: The Six Yogas of Naropa,' *Revolution of the Mind: Knowledge, Wisdom and Healing.* Proceedings of Rigpa Forum 1993. Barbara Lepani [ed.], Rigpa Australia Forum Publications. pp. 29-41, 142-143. Naropa,' *Revolution of the Mind: Knowledge, Wisdom and Healing.* Proceedings of Rigpa Forum

Stutchbury, Elisabeth, (1994a), 'Perceptions of Landscape in Karzha: Sacred Geography and the Tibetan System of Geomancy', *The Tibet Journal,* Vol. XIX, No. 4, pp. 59-102. Special edition, 'Powerful Places and Spaces in Tibetan Religious Culture', Antoni Huber [ed.].

Stutchbury, Elisabeth, (1994b), 'The Making of Gonpa: Norbu Rinpoche from Kardang and Kunga Rinpoche from Lama Gonpa.' In Samuel, G. B., H. Gregor and E. Stutchbury [eds.], *Tantra and Popular Religion in Tibet.* International Academy of Indian Culture and Aditya Prakashan, New Delhi. Sata-Pitaka Series Indo-Asian Literatures, Volume 376, pp. 155-204.

Stutchbury, Elisabeth, (Forthcoming a), *Rediscovering Western Tibet: Gonpa, Chorten and the Continuity of Practice With a Tibetan Buddhist Community in the Indian Himalaya.* State University of New York Press, McGill Studies in the History of Religion, Series Editor, Katherine K. Young. [PhD Dissertation].

Stutchbury, Elisabeth, (Forthcoming b), 'Dzogchen and Social Process - Transmission: Experience and Continuity in Tibetan Buddhism', in *Tibet in Context: Identity - Culture - History.* Edited by Elisabeth Stutchbury. Proceedings of Third Australasian Conference on Tibetan and Himalayan Studies.

Stutchbury, Elisabeth, (in press), 'Images of Change and Continuity in Karzha and the Ethnographic Mirror of the Sherpa in Nepal', in *Envisioning Tibet: People, Process and Practice.* Edited by Elisabeth Stutchbury and Hamish Gregor. Proceedings of Second Australasian Conference on Tibetan and Himalayan Studies. Aditya Prakashan. New Delhi.

Taylor, McComas, (1996 ms.) 'Did Alexandra David-Neel Ever Reach Lhasa?' Paper presented at in *Tibet in Context: Identity - Culture - History.* Third Australasian Conference on Tibetan and Himalayan Studies, RSPAS, ANU.

Thurman, Robert A. F., (1991), 'Tibetan Psychology: Sophisticated Software for the Human Brain', in Goleman & Thurman [eds.], pp. 53-73.

Thurman, Robert A. F., (1994), *The Tibetan Book of the Dead: Liberation Through Understanding in the Between.* New York, Aquarian/Bantam/Doubleday.

Tsering Lama Jampal Zangpo, (1988), *A Garland of Wish-fulfilling Trees. The Palyul Tradition of the*

Nyingmapa. Translated by Sangye Khandro. Ithaca, Snow Lion.

Vajradhatu Sun, (1981-1982), 'His Holiness in Zion, Illinios', Vol. 4, No. 2, p. 3.

Varela, Francesco J., Thompson, Evan & Rosch, Eleanor, (1993), *The Embodied Mind: Cognitive Science and Human Experience.* Cambridge Ma. & London, The MIT Press.

Wilber, Ken, (1977), *The Spectrum of Consciousness.* Illinios, Quest Books.

Wilber, Ken, [ed.], (1982), *The Holographic Paradigm and other Paradoxes: Exploring the Leading Edge of Science.* Boulder & London, New Science Library/Shambhala.

Wilber, Ken, (1983), *Eye to Eye: The Quest For the New Paradigm.* New York, Anchor/Doubleday.

Wodroffe, John, (1973), *The Serpent Power.* Madras, Ganesh & Co.

Yeshi Donden, (1986), *Health Through Balance: An Introduction To Tibetan Medicine.* Ithaca, Snow Lion.

Zukav, Gary, (1984), *The Dancing Wu Li Masters: An Overview of the New Physics.* London, Flamingo.

THE EMBODIED MIND, THE TALKING CURE AND THE SILENCE OF MEDITATION

Michael M. Del Monte, M.Sc., M.Psych.Sc., Ph.D.,
Senior Clinical Psychologist, St. Patrick's Hospital, Dublin, Ireland.

A Introduction:

In my previous introductory paper in this conference I discussed "the mind versus matter" debate as exemplified by the popularised view of Darwinian evolution. In it I cast doubts on any simplistic causal relationship between brain and mind. I go on in this paper to develop my contention that reality is experienced polymorphically at different levels along a concrete-abstract continuum. At the abstract, i.e. psychic, level the internal representations of reality are, to varying degrees, verbally labelled. However, this verbal symbolisation is rarely complete - even in adulthood, and hence the persistent need for somatisation.

This paper further goes on to examine, using constructivist and psychodynamic models, how verbalisation can be helpful in practice with psychosomatic and hysterical disorders. However, drawing on our understanding of meditation, the value of silence in psychotherapy for both patient and practitioner is discussed in the context of limitations to the "talking cure" - as verbalisation can be used as a higher order defense.

B. The Constructivist Approach

1. Reality

Allow me to return to the concept of polymorphic reality. Some authors contend that the world also can be dealt with at different levels of abstraction, i.e. from a concrete level to varying levels of subjective representations. Furthermore, George Kelly (1955) saw us as living in two realities - firstly the primary or external reality which lies beyond direct human perception, and secondly our interpretations or internal constructions of this primary reality. Likewise, Jaques Lacan (1966) theorised that we have to deal with three domains - the "real", the "imaginary" and the "symbolic", the latter two corresponding to Kelly's "internal constructions" and attempted communications thereof. For Kelly, we are like scientists developing "psychological constructs" (or hypotheses) in order to make sense of the world. These constructs, or discriminations, are initially pre-verbal (pre-linguistic) but the growing child comes to attach verbal labels to many such discriminations.

For Kelly our personal construct systems act as templates or "goggles" through which we perceive and experience the world. Thus, there is no fully objective perception of the world. As people move along the dimension of time they modify their personal constructions of reality so as to be able to anticipate more accurately the cutting edge of the present into the future. In a sense, construct systems are akin to personal "maps" that (ideally) are up-dated from time to time to produce a better fit with the external world (the "territory"). In other words, the construct systems of psychologically adapting individuals are constantly being revised in the light of newly assimilated evidence from an ever-changing world. Such psychological accommodation à la Piaget (1967) of our construct systems allows for a better fit with the flux of primary reality. However, such internal adjustments are far from straightforward, and are complicated by what we cannot readily comprehend and by what is not yet conscious.

2. The Unconscious

It is interesting to note the lay person's lack of enthusiasm for the Freudian concept of "the unconscious". Many go on referring to the "subconscious". This may be indicative of a preference for a concept which is more nuanced, less sharply delineated, i.e. less "black and white". Views of the "subconscious" tend to be confused with repressed material à la Freud (1912). Hence Kelly (1955) emphasized the importance of "*levels* of cognitive awareness". These levels of cognitive awareness can be seen as an elaboration of Freud's notion of the pre-conscious, but also as including layers within the unconscious. Others (e.g. Epstein, 1983) have followed Kelly's lead in emphasizing the importance of the pre-conscious.

3. The non-verbal domain

Kelly used the expression "pre-verbal construing" to cover a broad spectrum of sense-making which includes that which I would prefer to call non-verbal construing. Non-verbal constructs are those perceptual-emotional discriminations one makes which have not been verbally labelled. Consequently, they are often at a low level of cognitive awareness, and are largely sensed by us as "gut-feelings", intuitions, vague elusive sensations and fleeting impressions. They also include what Polanyi (1959) encompassed within the concept of "tacit knowledge" (as opposed to formal knowledge), and are typified by the phrase "we always know more than we can tell". For example, the tacit knowledge required to perform certain skills such as riding a bicycle is often more complex than we can express in terms of formal knowledge.

Knowledge (including memory) which has to be acted out in order to be communicated is usually at a relatively low level of cognitive awareness (as, for example, with those adults who were sexually abused in childhood but who have repressed or suppressed the memory thereof). Although non-verbal construing tends to represent a low level of awareness, it is not to be equated precisely with the unconscious. Some non-verbal construing may be communicated (often unknowingly or at the borders of consciousness) by means other than words, e.g. via behavioural "leakage". Such analogical communication stands in sharp contrast with the more usual verbal (or digital) communication. Analogical communication can also be conceptualized as psychological projection and is often picked up by its recipients as vague intuitions and so forth. When the recipient of such projections reciprocates in the prompted and desired manner, then we can describe this mutuality of feeling and behaviour as "projective identification". It can be an unconscious - or rather a "sub-conscious" mutuality. It is common in mother-infant relationships, among lovers and, of course, in psychotherapy dyads.

Pre-verbal constructs are those non-verbal constructs which have not yet been verbally labelled but which, in general, are capable of being so labelled. Insofar as many non-verbal constructs arise in pre-linguistic childhood and remain *poorly* verbalized (i.e. symbolized) they can also be referred to as sub-verbal constructs. When our sense-making discriminations become verbally labelled through speech they can be seen as cognitive (or verbal) constructs, whereas somatic construing tends to remain relatively unverbalised. Aspects of somatic construing include posture, balance, osmo-regulation and thermo-regulation.

Whilst some construing becomes formulated in symbolic speech, this is only the "tip of the iceberg". Much of non-verbal construing or discriminating can be seen in psycho-physiological terms having to do with phenomena such as pain, blood pressure responses, neuromuscular effects, endocrinological secretions, immune responses, gastro-intestinal reactions, kinaesthetics and the like. Such non-verbal processing has already been referred to as somatic construing. It literally plays a "vital" role in our self-organization. The sense-making of sub-human animals is largely or entirely confined to such somato-sensory construing (i.e. to proprioception, interoception and exteroception).

Ontogenetically (and phylogenetically) the "thinking-body" is developed out of the sensory and feeling body. This implies that imagery and feeling are primary to thinking (in the non-causal sense). In other words, in our evolutionary history we were perceiving and feeling creatures long before we acquired a capacity to think and speak. This developmental order also applies to our personal histories in that language skills take time to develop. In this way our personal history recapitulates our collective history.

In the absence of language a capacity for "hysterical" or collective identification allows groups of animals to behave as if they had a "group body-mind", e.g. shoals of fish, flocks of birds or sheep, and hives of bees and termites. In this way they can share perceptions and feelings - e.g. of danger. Humans, although retaining this capacity, do not need to rely on such "hysterical" identification in order to share feelings, i.e. to show "com-passion" or "sym-pathy". They learn to use language in a social context. In order to talk about experiences (e.g. feelings of anger, envy or nausea) we need to use verbal labels. ("Putting verbal form on feelings"). The usage of such labels means that much primary sense-making acquires a secondary, i.e. cognitive or abstract overlay.

Incidentally, the Kellian dialectic of pre-verbal construing versus cognitive construing has considerable overlap with the Freudian dichotomy of primary process versus secondary process mentation. Kelly sees the individual as initially constructing his or her own reality at the pre-verbal level and then increasingly going on to construct a sense of reality at the level of (social) linguistic symbolism - namely by developing cognitive constructs (or secondary process cognition in Freudian terms). Hence, the "talking body" is emergent out of a sensory-affective condition in a social context. In evolutionary terms both projective and "hysterical" identification, as well as "languaging", are adaptive insofar as they facilitate communication, the difference being that speech operates at an abstract level of symbolism and represents an adaptation into the "Symbolic Order" à la Lacan.

4. Somatic Disorders

There can be problems in the development of symbolisation. We can thus turn to the field of psychosomatic and hysterical disorders where complaints are largely manifested in the somatic format. Patients with psychosomatic symptoms tend to be very concrete in their presentation of complaints due to a difficulty with verbal symbolisation. In discussing disorders involving psychosomatic symptoms, Kelly illustrates how the "mind-body" construct can be applied pre-emptively by such patients. This is where people often show a strong "mind-body" split. The difficulty lies in concrete and dualistic thinking. The person is unable to construe herself as a whole because the body is construed in a "mechanical" manner and the area of mind is construed largely in a separate "intellectualized" way (Kelly, 1955, p.921). A solution, according to Kelly, for overcoming such mind/body dualism is to be found in (adaptive) regression to early forms of pre-verbal thinking - "Only at that primitive level may we find that the mind and the body were not pre-emptively separated". There are several pathways to achieving such adaptive regression - such as psychotherapy, psycho-analysis, meditation and hypnosis.

As already mentioned, pre-verbal constructs originated mostly in infancy in order to make sense of those elements of life encountered by the infant in its growth and development. When people get into difficulty using their adult constructions, their last line of "defence" is often mal-adaptive regression to the pre-verbal constructions of infancy, with its attendant infantile dependency. Hence we often find psychosomatic symptomatology accompanying strong unfulfilled dependency needs. Hysterical symptomatology, likewise associated with dependency needs, often symbolizes strong unconscious conflicts, which one defensively avoids because of inherent feelings of shame or guilt.

The psycho-analyst Hogan (1995) presents an interesting comparison between hysterical somatoform conversions, which he sees as post-oedipally symbolic, and the more primitive pre-oedipal psychosomatic disorders which, he claims, operate at a lower (i.e. often pre-verbal) level of symbolism, with less conscious control. For Hogan, psychosomatic disease of the gut can either represent psychosexual developmental arrest at the oral-anal (i.e. "gut") phase, or an emotional regression back to that phase following a perceived threat to one's security. In this respect Hogan sees the alexithymia of many psychosomatic patients as a defence against the shame felt about negative fantasies and feelings by blocking their conscious verbalisation. Instead these negative impulses are directed inwards to produce "masochistic gratification in the pain of psychosomatic symptoms". This masochism, coupled with alexithymia and/or other defensive postures, makes psychosomatic disorders difficult to treat. So it is to treatment issues that we now turn.

5. Abreaction, insight and integration

It has been argued by McGee, et al. (1984) that emotional experiences which are too threatening to one's core psychological functioning can be defensively suspended as "un-experienced experiences", i.e. without being fully processed or integrated at a cognitive and conscious level. In this sense, such experiences remain akin to the "unfinished business", the "unfulfilled needs", or the "incomplete Gestalten" referred to by Gestalt therapists. These incomplete Gestalten are usually at low levels of awareness and tend to be projected or "acted out" behaviourly, e.g. hysterically, in order to be communicated (- often with considerable feeling but with little thought). In this sense the symptoms of hysteria are seen to be functional and symbolic (Szasz, 1972). The weakening of one's emotional defences during psychotherapy facilitates the abreactive emergence of such incomplete Gestalten and other repressed material. In other words, the experience which was held in a sort of "suspended animation" can be relived emotionally - initially as "somatic memory", then with hindsight reprocessed and integrated into one's personal construct system at a more insightful level of awareness.

Such integration or assimilation of past experiences into a construct system can be envisaged as requiring cognitive accommodation in the Piagetian sense (Piaget, 1967). This accommodation usually leads to a tighter (cognitive) understanding of the largely sub-verbal experiences had during cathartic abreaction and should enable the client to put some verbal structure onto these pre-verbal feelings. By learning to put verbal form on feeling, the client is in a better position to discuss his or her experiences with others - including the therapist. She can also "save" energy heretofore required to repress those psychodynamically threatening events relived during abreaction. I shall next look at the role of therapists in such treatment dyads.

6. Therapeutic Attention

Allow me to continue with some classical quotations. Freud stated that a psycho-analyst should maintain an "evenly hovering attention" between patient and self in the selection of material during analysis, but "if one's expectations are followed in this selection, there is the danger of never finding anything but what is already known" (Freud, 1912, pp.111-112). To my knowledge Freud did not go on to describe how this important advice could be cultivated. Did Bion (1970) take him up when he advised analysts to forsake "memory, desire and understanding" during practice? By suggesting that analysts eschew these three functions was Bion reformulating Freud's original advice not to follow one's expectations in therapy? In a similar vein Bion quoted from a letter by John Keats, written in 1817, in which Keats referred to "Negative Capability" as "when a man is capable of being in uncertainties, mysteries, doubts, without any irritable reaching after fact and reason" (Bion, 1970, p.125). It is my hope that a deeper understanding of meditative silence will allow us to address, later on, the issues just raised by my quotations from Freud and Bion. Bion was perhaps one of the most mystical of all psycho-analysts and it is thus to mysticism that we now turn.

C. Relevance of Meditation and Mysticism

1. Mysticism

Let me continue with a paradox. Ria Weyens stated, "We are afraid of the void" (Weyens, 1992). Yet she also said that "emptiness is the source of fullness", and that to develop fullness "We must find the no-self or selfless-self". To help resolve the above paradoxes it is useful to look at the tradition of mysticism. Mysticism, like psychoanalysis, is a quest into the unknown. For Louth (1992) it is more likely to be characterised by the workings of Eros than by Logos. Hence according to Louth the unknowable reality of God cannot be logically apprehended, but is experienced by "transformation of the soul" via Eros. (Eros may be conceptually similar to the vital energy, Yuan Shen, of Qi-gong).

Mysticism is thus concerned with transcending our habitual dualistic construing of the world. According to Stace (1960) mysticism has to do with the essential unity of experience, e.g. "the seer and the seen are one". Techniques used to gain access to the experience of this unity include yoga, Qi-gong and meditation. With these techniques practitioners regularly report that the usual dimensions of time and space become perceptually distorted - often accompanied by an upsurge of emotion - sometimes referred to as "unstressing" (DelMonte, 1990).

Mysticism has two main approaches - the "via positiva" and the "via negativa". The former, based more on logic and objectivity, tends to focus on what the practitioner gains from the mystical experience. The via negativa, on the contrary, is concerned with emptiness, void and nothingness and tolerance thereof. Bion's views on "negative capability" come to mind here.

In meditation, by focusing exclusively and continuously on *one* meaningless stimulus (e.g. a mantra), all contrasts fall away. As contrasts are necessary for ordinary sense-making one is left with ***nothing*** to construe or "no-thought" (see DelMonte, 1987). This is the nothingness of the via negativa. Sustained "nothingness" can lead to an ineffable transcendental state of non-attachment and equanimity, in which one experiences undifferentiated unity, i.e. the Infinite or God (see DelMonte, 1995). This is just one example of how meditation is embedded in mysticism and spirituality.

2. The role of silence

Psychotherapy, compared with meditation, is a neophyte on the world stage. Most forms of psychotherapy use verbalisation as their modus operandi. A common view held by psycho-analysts is that those who do not learn to "think" (i.e. to symbolise abstractly) are bound to go on suffering - as with hysterics who "feel" too much. While one would not dispute that there is great merit in the "talking cure" approach there is, nevertheless, a growing corpus of opinion on the value of silence in therapy. For example, obsessionals, in thinking and talking too much, demonstrate "the negative power of thinking". In therapy they typically have difficulty in being in touch with feelings - their own and those of others - and are usually very uncomfortable with silence. Hence the endless chatter - often split off from feeling. This is sometimes referred to as "free dissociation" (Perls, et al., 1973) or split-off intellect. These people need to learn that speech, like music, is given deeper meaning by being punctuated by silence.

Silence on the part of the patient was seen as resistance by Freud (1912). However, Balint (1958) argued that "if we can change our own approach - from considering silence as a symptom of resistance to studying it as a possible *source of information* - then we may learn something about this area of mind". Later authors saw silence as indicative of shyness, shame, sorrow, anger, hostility, psychic absence and fear (Shafii, 1973; Coltart, 1992). Silence has also been construed, at times, as adaptive regression to preverbal sense-making (as opposed to malign or psychotic regression - Shafii, 1973), or the unconscious need for "total union with mother" (Shafii, 1973).

In keeping with this theme Shafii (1973) sees words as creating communication, and silence as fostering communion. The psychoanalyst Coltart (1992) goes as far as saying that "my own preference, above all others, is for a silent patient". This may be because the relatively silent patient allows the analyst ample time to work with the visceral felt-sense of the counter-transference. It should come as no surprise that Coltart also describes herself as a practitioner of meditation and Buddhism. This is a long way from Freud who did not work with the counter-transference, and who saw religious experience, meditation and mysticism as regressive and mal-adaptive phenomena, i.e. forms of oceanic fusion and oneness with mother, or the wish to re-experience intra-uterine life (Freud, 1930). To facilitate the patient in adaptive regression the therapist must also be capable of silence, e.g. by avoiding premature, aggressive and excessive interpretations or comments. In this way pre-verbal traumata can be "re-experienced and mastered again in silence" (Shafii, 1973). There are probably several ways in which therapists can learn to be comfortable with silence. One pathway is via meditation.

3. Meditation and the psychotherapist

Many authors have written on how the practice of meditation by psychotherapists can enhance receptivity, empathy, staying in the "hic et nunc" (here and now), and the use of counter-transference (Lesh, 1970; Carrington & Ephron, 1975; Keefe, 1975; Speeth, 1982; Rubin, 1985; DelMonte, 1987, 1990; Coltart, 1992). For example, Speeth argued cogently that meditation can be a form of attention training. She sees that concentrative meditation is a training in narrowly focused or specifically invested attention, whereas mindfulness meditation trains one to adopt a non-attached, panoramic or wide-focus attention, which is evenly invested in everything that comes to mind - namely a kind of "choiceless awareness". Allied to these two approaches Speeth also describes a third (and higher) level of integrated attention which she calls "witness consciousness". This involves an awareness of the type of attention being given (narrow or panoramic), as well as the object of attention. Is this "witness consciousness" similar to Freud's "evenly hovering attention"? Bion's advice to forsake "memory, desire and understanding" when listening to patients also comes to mind here.

In a similar vein, Rubin (1985) argued that training in both concentrative and mindfulness meditation enhances "psychoanalytic listening". He postulated that meditation produces a "laying fallow" state of mind. Such a state would be more receptive to any pregnant silence emergent from the analytic dyad. Fromm (1977), in an excellent article, descriptively contends that the practice of meditation helps to make the unconscious conscious by enhancing ego receptivity, primary process mentation, fantasy, imagery, free-floating attention and adaptive regression. Finally, on this theme, Coltart (1992) argues that since much of what patients present to us is "beyond words" (as in psychosomatic symptoms and hysterical conversions) it cannot simply be dealt with at the level of language. Instead she uses her training in meditation to enhance neutral or "bare attention", both "sharply focused and scanning" to tune into the patient's transferences, and especially, into her own counter-transference. It is worth quoting her conclusion on this subject. "The discipline of meditation practice enhances the discipline of one's contribution to an analytic session which sometimes is, in fact, itself almost indistinguishable from a form of meditation" (p.147). I would call this mindfulness. Such mindfulness aids attunement with both the patient and one's own counter-transference.

All of this is not to argue that during therapy, patient and therapist must sit out session after session in blissful silence! Rather, the *ability* to suspend, at critical moments, the complex cognitive processes involved in "memory, desire and understanding" (Bion) is a stance in therapy which meditation training enhances. It is not so much a question of forsaking or eschewing memory and desire like Bion advised, but rather temporarily holding them in abeyance. This is precisely what mindfulness meditation is all about. This process has also been referred to as the "de-automatization" of cognitive construing (Fromm, 1977; DelMonte & Kenny, 1985; DelMonte, 1987, 1990), and is akin to Bion's use of the expression "negative capability", which, as already mentioned, refers to the therapist,s capacity to suspend logic and dwell in uncertainties, mysteries and doubts. Hence we can conceptually link Bion's "negative capability" and Freud's "evenly hovering attention" to the mindfulness fostered by meditation.

4. Critique and Conclusions

Most schools of meditation have little to say about finding, owning and coming to terms with our inner "badness" or destructiveness (e.g. anger, hatred, lust, envy and the like). Zen Buddhists refer to "Makyo" as morbid, unwanted, unconscious material which interferes with meditation by arising spontaneously during its practice (Russell, 1986). Meditation instructors usually do not seek to analyse emergent makyo. In this respect the practice of traditional meditation differs from psychotherapy. With the latter, there is an attempt to integrate split off goodness (ego-ideals and idealised objects) and badness (our "shadows") rather than "side-stepping" our unwanted parts (see Main, 1982, 1984, 1989; DelMonte 1995). Psycho-analysts see splitting as weakening the ego. The approach in meditation is to move beyond the dictate of the ego. A difficulty with this approach could be that individuals who have rather fragmented egos tend to be drawn to meditation, yet may experience considerable difficulty in transcending their unintegrated egos. Paradoxically, we need reasonably good "ego-strength" to help us transcend those ego strivings that temporarily yield some pleasure but ultimately little happiness. Hence such transcendence depends for its success on a healthy ego being able to temporarily suspend its functioning (DelMonte, 1987, 1990, 1995).

Another worry is that schizoid or "split-off" individuals may use meditation as a defense to escape even further from the world, and rather than feeling "connected" they may become even more dissociated and cut off from others. Meditation is no substitute for psychotherapy but rather can supplement it, especially for those who have gained sufficient ego-strength.

A problem with those who exclusively advocate the "via negativa" is that they tend to deify the "no-self" or "nothingness" experience. Although such experience can have enormous spiritual value for some it can also be a defensive escape into "narcissistic emptiness" (Epstein, 1990). In other words, there can be a confusion between egolessness and self-abnegation. The latter has been described as pathological de-personalisation and de-realisation, i.e. hysterical dissociation (Castillo, 1990). Meditation can be used to deny the existence of body and aspects of external reality, thereby increasing splits such as found in "mind/body" and "person/world" (i.e. subject/object) dualism. Worse still there is the risk that the via negativa can turn into a painless form of premature self-destruction anticipating death, i.e. working more in the service of thanatos than of eros.

As already suggested some people may turn to meditation as a defense by using it to distance themselves from what they regard as unworthy parts of themselves - namely their aggression, sexuality, intellect, envy and so forth. But, as Epstein points out, these functions are still present (only denied). "Such people often find themselves irresistibly attracted to powerful others who come to contain essential ego functions that are otherwise disavowed" (Epstein, 1990, p.78). Hence the cult leader phenomenon. This tendency is also found with respect to popular dictators.

The path of meditation (silence) should not seek to destroy the embodied ego, but rather to accomplish the liberation of self from blind allegiance to impulses and from the impoverishment resulting from our defenses. Meditation should allow ego just to be ego - neither permanently subjected to repudiation per la via negativa nor indulged with narcissistic grandiosity. The insights gained through psychotherapy show us that Eros cannot stand alone without Thanatos, and that the via negativa, without the bridle of logic afforded by the via positiva, may be no more than an elaborate defense.

Finally, the conclusions of this paper may appear rather paradoxical. Having initially argued for the value of the "talking cure" in dealing with psychosomatic and hysterical disorders by learning to put verbal form on elusive feelings, I then go on to deconstruct the notion that such verbalisation be seen as a clinical panacea. Here the value of silence in therapy, as exemplified by meditation, is also acknowledged. There are limits to the "talking cure". Learning to put verbal form on feelings can be developmentally liberating, but can also be defensive - as with intellectualisation, mis-attribution and rationalisation - which serve to contort and reframe the truth of our emotional underworlds. Hence simplistic notions that mind is superior to body, that "abstract" is better than "concrete" or that one "causes" the other, are just dualistic fallacies! Beyond both matter and mind, i.e. beyond body and language, lies the ineffable domain beyond symbolisation - namely stillness and silence. Cultivation of silence allows one to pay attention to feelings. Emotions are the connection between mind and body, and thus can play an integrative role. So we end this paper near to where we began, by allusion to that realm variously described as "the real", "primary reality" or that extra-linguistic domain so feared, and yet so desired, by us.

References

1. Balint, M. (1958). The three areas of the mind. *International Journal of Psycho-Analysis*, 39, 328-340.
2. Bion, W.R. (1970). *Attention and Interpretation*, Tavistock, London.
3. Carrington, P. & Ephron, H. Meditation and Psychoanalysis (1975b) *Journal of the American Academy of Psychoanalysis*, 3(i), 43-57.
4. Castillo, R.J. (1990). Depersonalization and Meditation. *Psychiatry*, 53, 158-168.
5. Coltart, N. (1992). *Slouching Towards Bethlehem: And Further Psychoanalytic Explorations*. Free Association Books, London.
6. DelMonte, M.M. (1987). A constructivist view of meditation. *American Journal of Psychotherapy*, 41(2), 286-298.
7. DelMonte, M.M. (1990). The relevance of meditation to clinical practice: An overview. *Applied Psychology: An International Review*. 39(3), 331-354.
8. DelMonte, M.M. (1995). Silence and emptiness in the service of healing: Lessons from Meditation. *British Journal of Psychotherapy*, 11(3), 368-378.
9. DelMonte, M.M. & Kenny, V. (1985). Models of Meditation. *British Journal of Psychotherapy*, 1(3), 197-214.
10. Epstein, M. (1990). Psychodynamics of meditation: Pitfalls on the spiritual path. *Journal of Transpersonal Psychology*, 22(1), 17-34.
11. Epstein, S. (1983). The unconscious, the pre-conscious, and self-concept. In J. Suls and A.G. Greenwald (Eds.), *Psychological Perspectives of the self*, Vol.2, L.E.A. Publishers, London, pp.291-247.
12. Freud, S. (1912). *Recommendations to Physicians Practising Psycho-Analysis*: Standard Edition, 12, 111-120. Hogarth Press, London, 1955.
13. Freud, S. (1930). *Civilisation and its Discontents*, Standard Edition, Hogarth Press, London.
14. Fromm, E. (1977). An ego-psychological theory of altered states of consciousness. *International Journal of Clinical and Experimental Hypnosis*, 25(4), 372-387.
15. Hogan, C.C. (1995). *Psychosomatics, Psychoanalysis and Inflammatory Disease of the Colon*: International Universities Press; Madison, Connecticut.
16. Jung, C. (1958). Psychological commentary on the Tibetan book of the great liberation. In *Psychology and Religion, Vol.2 Collected Works*, Pantheon Books, New York.
17. Keefe, T. (1975). Meditation and the Psychotherapist. *American Journal of Orthopsychiatry*, 45(3), 484-489.
18. Kelly, G.A. (1955). *The Psychology of Personal Constructs*, Norton, New York.
19. Lacan, J. (1966). *Ecrits*, Senils, Paris.
20. Lesh. T.V. (1970). Zen Meditation and the development of empathy in counsellors. *Journal of*

Humanistic Psychology, 10, 39-74.

21. Louth, A. (1992). Eros and Mysticism. *The Guild of Pastoral Psychology*, Guild Lecture No.241, London.
22. McGee, D.; Brown, I.; Kenny V.; McGennis, A. & Pilot, J. (1984). Unexperienced experience: A critical reappraisal of the theory of regression and traumatic neurosis. *Irish Journal of Psychotherapy*, 3 (1), 7-19.
23. Main, J. (1982). *Letters from the Heart*, Crossroads, New York.
24. Main, J. (1984). *Moment of Christ: The Path of Meditation*, Darton, Longman & Todd, London.
25. Main, J. (1989). *The Way of Unknowing*. Darton, Longman & Todd, London.
26. Perls, F.S., Hefferline, R.F., & Goodman, P. (1973). *Gestalt Therapy: Excitement and Growth in the Human Personality*, Penguin, London.
27. Piaget, J. (1967). *The Psychology of Intelligence*, Routledge Kegan Paul, London.
28. Polanyi, M. (1959). *The Study of Man*, University of Chicago Press, Chicago.
29. Rubin, J.B. (1985). Meditation and psychoanalytic listening. *Psychoanalytic Review*, 72(4), 599-613.
30. Russell, E.W. (1986). Consciousness and the unconscious: Eastern meditative and Western therapeutic approaches. *Journal of Transpersonal Psychology*, 18(1), 51-72.
31. Shafii, M. (1973). Silence in the service of the ego: Psychoanalytic study of meditation. *International Journal of Psychoanalysis*, 54(4), pp.431-443.
32. Speeth, K.R. (1982). On therapeutic attention. *Journal of Transpersonal Psychology*, 14(2), 141-160.
33. Stace, W.T. (1960). *The Teachings of the Mystics*, Mentor, New York.
34. Szasz, T.S. (1972). *The Myth of Mental Illness*, Paladin, London.
35. Teilhard de Chardin, P. (1965). *The Phenomenon of Man*, Fontana, London.
36. Weyens, R. (1992). Lectio Divina. In. *Proceedings of the Workshop: Towards the Whole Person: Integrating Eastern and Western Approaches to Body-Mind Skills*, St. Andries Benedictine Abbey, Brugge, 15th-17th July, pp.48-51.

PART II

SYMPOSIUM ORGANISED BY THE TRANS-NATIONAL NETWORK FOR THE STUDY OF PHYSICAL, PSYCHOLOGICAL AND SPIRITUAL WELL-BEING, HELD AT THE 26TH INTERNATIONAL CONGRESS OF PSYCHOLOGY, ENTITLED: "DOES THE CONCEPT OF EMBODIMENT OFFER SOMETHING NEW IN PSYCHOLOGY?

Yutaka Haruki and Jon Kabat-Zinn, Convenors and Chairmen
Yutaka Haruki and Michael DelMonte, Editors

20th August 1996

Montreal
Canada

EMBODIED MIND AND "MINI SHIMITE WAKARU"

Opening Address for the Symposium on "Does the Concept of Embodiment Offer Something New in Psychology?" at the XXVI International Congress of Psychology, Montreal,
Yutaka Haruki, Ph. D., Professor of Psychology, Waseda University, Japan

The subject on the relationship between mind and body has always been a subject of interest and debate from ancient times. The understanding of the relationship between the two has been greatly influenced by Descartes' body and mind dualism. In other words, it is understood that the mind and the body are two different existences. Modern medicine has made rapid advances and achieved a remarkable success by separating the elements of the mind from the body and adhereing to the theory that the body is a material object or a substance. The mind, separated from the body, has been treated as an isolated subject. Namely, problems of the body have been attributed to be caused by the body and problems of the mind to be caused by the mind. The relationship between the two is as illustrated in 1 and 2 of the diagram.

Other than coming up with the theory that mind and body are two separate things, studies have been done with respect to the interactions between the two. For example, brain physiologists have shed much light on the relationship between certain areas of the cerebral cortex and mental activities. The development of molecular biology has helped to clarify the relationship between material objects and mental activities. Psychopharmacological drugs represent one of these successful achievements.

On the other hand, it has become clear pari passu with the development of psychosomatic medicine and health psychology that the mind affects the body. We might expect psychoneuroimmunology to soon clarify the mechanism of the relationship between mind and body. These relationships are as shown in 3 and 4 of the diagram. It may be said that some recent topics of scientific studies are useful in considering the relationship between mind and body.

In considering the relationship between mind and body, there may be two paradigms. One of them, as shown in 3 of the diagram, is the study of the mind in the context of the body and the other, as shown in 4 of the diagram, is the study of the body in the context of the mind. Biologists and physiologists who are pursuing the studies of the body usually study the mind in the context of the body. On the contrary, philosophers and psychologists tend to consider the body in the context of the mind. It is generally believed unusual for biologists to consider the body in the context of the mind and for psychologists to consider the mind in the context of the body. This is basically because Descartes' mind and body dualism concerning human beings has suppressed the freedom of our thought. Human beings are not made of mind and body. Rather, human beings make up body and mind. The thought that human beings consist of mind and body is merely an outgrowth of the idea resulting from such recognition. This means we are free to think any way we want with respect to the relationship between the two.

I'd like to discuss the matter within the context of psychology. Recognizing a human being as "mind", and studying the effects of the mind on the body have been a traditional pattern of the study of psychology. In contrast, we'd like to think about how the body is related to the mind and how the mind is studied from the perspective of the body. The study of the mind in the context of the body as an object material has been made in the fields of brain physiology and psychopharmacology. However, little psychological study has been made based on this paradigm. When we think of the body in the context of psycology, the body is not a body as a material object, but the sensibility of a body, a movement of a body and an act of a body. In other words, it is something to be experienced by a body. The mind without the body would be nothing more than an abstract concept. Therefore, the mind embodied in such a body may be described in fact as the mind of an actually existing human being. Little basic study has been made based on this paradigm. This has been put into practice in the field of psychotherapy, however. Body-work is a good example case. The mechanism concerning its psychological effects has yet to be clarified.

"Wakaru"1) and "mini shimite wakaru"2) are Japanese words. "Wakaru" means to understand the logic of a language. In other words, it means to understand something with the mind. "Mini shimite wakaru" means not only to understand something with logic but with feelings or emotions. In other words, it means to understand something with bodily experience. As for the way we human beings are actually made, the mind permeates the body and the body permeates the mind. So, this is what I think. To really "understand" something means to "understand" something with mind and body.

There may be a great many difficulties in the study of the relationship between body and mind, but the study of an embodied mind is expected to open a new horizen for

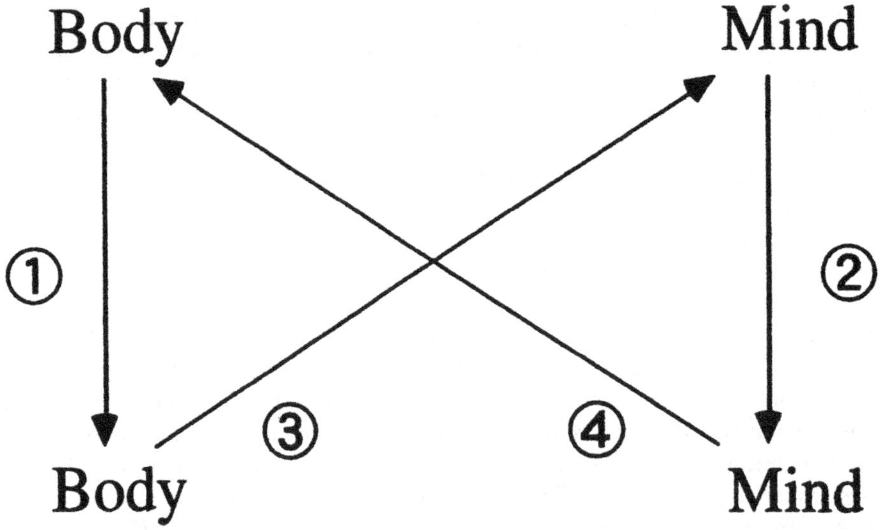

Mind/Body relationship

resolving problems on mind within the context of psychology. This trend can be seen in recent works such as F. J. Varela et al (Eds) "The embodied mind" and M. J. Mahoney "Embodying the mind; Incorporating the body into psychotherapy" (in press). I hope this symposium represents a step forward in that direction.

Foot Note:

1) Wakaru: Understand

2) Mini: bodily Shimite: permeate, infiltrate into Mini shimite wakaru: understand deeply or really

THE MATTER OF MIND: EMOTIONS AS THE MIND-BODY CONNECTION

Candace B. Pert, PhD,
Research Professor, Department of Physiology &Biophysics, Georgetown University, School of Medicine, Washington DC, U.S.A.

THE DISEMBODIED BRAIN

I am a "neuroscientist", having begun to study the brain 25 years ago, when this term was newly coined for a brand new interdisciplinary field. I entered neuroscience because I was interested in consciousness, and I assumed that consciousness was in the brain. That's why I began to study the brain, and little did I know that the assumption that the mind is inside the brain..would prove wrong.... A definition of mind which seems to predominate in Western culture is "a control system implemented in brain." My laboratory research---which has been accepted and replicated all over the world-- has led to the realization that this assumption is WRONG! It is disembodied, and I used to be disembodied myself. For many years at the NIH outside of Washington, DC, I worked in the Brain Biochemistry Section, which I had founded to map the brain which I thought was "it", the end-all and be-all of consciousness.

Even though I have worked for years in the mecca of mainstream medicine, I am much less enthusiastic about its "breakthroughs" and progress than most doctors and even scientists. In fact, I believe that mainstream medicine has come to an impenetrable wall, for so many chronic diseases there is really no help. Cancer, of course, is foremost in this category in terms of the amount of funds and energy that have been expended with minimal results, eg almost all forms of chemotherapy available today were invented prior to 1960! I believe that this has occurred because we are stuck in an outdated, erroneous paradigm that sees health as good functioning of a billion tiny pieces and sees diseases as broken parts that can be fixed or replaced. Until we address the real nature of human beings---they are not disembodied brains attached to a life support system otherwise known as their bodies!--- we will not progress any further in curing cancer or any other chronic diseases which seem to be increasing in frequency at the same time we are supposedly making more "breakthroughs" by decoding more genes.

EMOTIONS: THE MIND – BODY CONNECTION

My colleague Michael Ruff and I defined "psychoimmunoendocrine network" in our 1984 *Science* paper, the idea of an information network being composed of neuropeptides and receptors. The key was the realization that the same molecules are communicating to join all of these systems of the body into one unit, the bodymind; with the notable exceptions of the steroid sex hormones and the amino acid-based and -derived neurotransmitters, these molecules are peptides. In 1985, in a special August supplement of the *Journal of Immunology* , we theorized, based upon several newly discovered facts, in an article entitle "Neuropeptides and Their Receptors: The Psychosomatic Network", that neuropeptides and their receptors are the biochemical basis of our emotions. So we visualize emotions as the the interplay of peptides and other ligands or information molecules (a term coined initially by F.O. Schmitt) with their receptors.

Our group came to hypothesize that these chemicals, neuropeptides and their receptors, are biological substrates of emotions when we found receptors for 70-80 peptide substances in the amygdala, the hypothalamus, and other areas of the brain that were classically thought to mediate emotions. Another key line of reasoning that led to this theory is that peptide ligands and their receptors remain stable across millions of years of evolution, just as Charles Darwin predicted for the physiological components of emotions, which he saw as so essential to survival that they would have evolved early and be passed on and conserved. Even the simplest of organisms, one-celled creatures like yeast and Tetrahymena contain endorphins and insulin and have opiate receptors and insulin receptors on their cellular surface. Interestingly, anxiety seems to be a rather advanced emotion, since the "anxiety peptide" which binds to the valium/librium receptor can only be found in more recently evolved creatures like the bony fish (teleosts) and beyond. Finally, the fact that all psychoactive drugs---which alter mood and state of consciousness -- work by plugging into receptors meant for internal ligands shows that the natural information network, spanning brain and body, gives us feelings as it runs the physiology.

Receptors and their ligands

The first component of the molecules of emotion is a cellular mechanism called the opiate receptor. It was the discovery of the opiate receptor which launched my career as a bench scientist in the early 70's, when I devised a method to measure it – thereby proving that it did indeed exist – for the very first time. But what is a receptor?

At the time I was getting started, a receptor was mostly an idea, a hypothetical site believed to be located somewhere in the cells of all living things. The scientists who most needed to believe in it were the pharmacologists because they were trying to explain the action of drugs in the organism.

Dating back to the early 20th century, pharmacologists believed that each and every drug acting in the body must first attach itself by means of something called a receptor, a mechanism that would allow it to enter the cell. This attachment of the drug to the receptor, called binding, occurred in a mysterious way and was thought to initiate a cascade of physiological changes. "No drug acts unless it is fixed," said Paul Erlich, the first pharmacologist, summarizing what he believed to be true, even though he had no real evidence. Except he said it in Latin to emphasize the profundity of the concept.

Now we know that a receptor is a single molecule, perhaps the most elegant, rare and complicated kind of molecule there is. A molecule is the tiniest possible piece of a substance that can still be identified as that substance. Composing each and every molecule of any given substance are the smallest units of matter, atoms like carbon and hydrogen and nitrogen, which are identically bonded together in a configuration which can be written by a chemical formula, or more informatively, drawn as a diagram.

Invisible forces attract one molecule to another, eventually making up the cohesive substance. These invisible forces of attraction can be overcome if enough energy is applied to the substance. For example, heat energy will melt ice crystals, turning them into water, which will then vaporize into steam as its molecules move so fast, with so much energy, that they break loose of each other and fly apart. Water still has the same chemical formula, H2O, two hydrogen atoms bonded to one oxygen atom, whether it is an icy solid, a watery liquid or a colorless vapor.

In contrast to the small, rigid water molecule, which weighs only 18 units in molecular weight, the larger receptor molecule weighs upwards of 50,000 units. Unlike the water molecule that flies apart when energy is applied, the more flexible receptor molecule responds by vibrating, instead of melting or turning into a gas. They wiggle, shimmy and even hum as they bend and change from one shape to another, often going back and forth between two or three favored shapes or conformations. Unless a receptor has been purified in the lab from some creature's tissues, you'd never find one by itself, with no other substances present. In the organism, they are always found attached to a cell, sitting on the surface wall with their roots enmeshed in the cell's oily, outer boundary, called the membrane, snaking back and forth across it several times.

Most of the cells in our bodies are studded with hundreds of thousands of receptors, crowded together like so many lillypads floating on a large shallow lake. But unlike lillypads, whose roots anchor the whole plant, keeping it fixed to one spot, receptors can slide anywhere along the surface of the cell membrane. The activity of the cell at any given moment, whether it's dividing or not dividing, cooking up biochemicals or not (these are some of the things cells do), is influenced by two things: What particular receptors populate its surface and what kind of shape they have assumed – how they're humming, so to speak.

What causes the receptors to do their little song and dance? The responsible element is called a ligand, which is a term used to cover any number of substances from neurotransmitters, through peptides to steroids like estrogen. All that is required of a substance to be classified as a ligand is that it binds to a receptor, seeming to enter it like a key into a lock, creating a perturbence to tickle the molecules into rearranging themselves, changing their shape and – click! – opening a doorway into the cell. What a cell is doing every moment, whether it has decided to divide or not to divide and form two new cells, whether it will make this protein or stop making that protein depends on how many of the cell's receptors are occupied by their specific ligands at that moment.

Using the modern biomolecular techniques available today, scores of new receptors are being cloned and sequenced, meaning that their complete chemical structure can now be diagramed.

The psychosomatic network

I'm glad I touched on some chemistry , because you need to appreciate the chemistry to grok the truth about the newly emergent field some have called "psychoneuroimmunology" and how your emotions run every system of your body.. The key aspect is that the bodymind (yes, there's no hyphen, one word) must be viewed in its holistic entirety. Just because universities like to separate departments of immunology from departments of neuroscience for traditional and political reasons, doesn't mean the bodymind doesn't have all systems intimately connected by the cross hum of ligands, informational substances and peptides binding to their receptors.

I actually detest the word psychoneuroimmunology, probably because I didn't think of it first. No, there are some legitimate reasons for hating it. It's so apologetic as far as psycho- is concerned--it quickly adds neuro- as if psycho- is too unscientific on its own. But it's inaccurate to single out neuro- when the peptide-providing glial cells of the brain are at least as as important as the neurons, nurturing them as they secrete numerous peptide ligands that literarily "make up your mind", sculpting the connections or synapses between one neuron and another and acting as "growth factors". Psychoneuroimmunology leaves out endocrinology and hence loses a key idea---that the brain is a great big ductless gland chock full of neuropeptide hormones coming out of glial cells and neurons in the brain, entering from the body and going everywhere.

In 1988, the cover of Newsweek magazine, deeply shocked, upset, and troubled the scientists like myself who were interviewed for a wonderful article on the emerging science called "psychoneuroimmunology". Somehow the editors of the popular newsmagazine had chosen to place the four-letter word "Soul" right on its cover next to that deliberately jargony, safe, multisyllabic term often abbreviated "PNI". Soul is not a word used in science, even though it is the root word for psychology. Descartes had excised the concept of soul, mind and emotions out of science, psychology and Western thought a few hundred years ago when he struck a turf deal with the Pope. These abstract concepts would stay in the realm of the Church, and in return, Descartes was allowed access to dissect the cadavers that he needed to lay the foundation of what later became modern biochemistry – the whole as broken down, reduced into its billion parts to be studied separately from each other and certainly with mind and emotions excluded from the mix. The mind-body split needs to be healed in light of recent scientific discoveries which show that the molecules of mind and emotion are inseparable from the physiology of the body. I am convinced that it must be healed to produce a new paradigm before diseases can be cured.

Emotions, reality, consciousness health and disease

Not only are emotions the bridge between mind and body, I believe--extrapolating from research findings-- that emotions are the bridge between mind and matter in general. Emotions occupy both realms, the spiritual and the physical--and they may be the transforming principle between the two. In the body, they are in the form of actual molecules that have been evolving for millions of years. In the spiritual realm, emotions are the glue that bonds interpersonal relationships --or drives them apart.

The anatomical distribution pattern of neuropeptides and their receptors---being enriched in several "nodal points" like the dorsal horn of the spinal cord and other sensory input areas-- suggests that all sensations and perceptions are filtered through our emotions. Not just primary somatosensory input into the brain, but even sight, sound, smell, taste and touch are filtered through a gradient of these informational substances and their receptors. Each person's perceptions, sensations and hence reality is different, based upon the conditioning that has occurred because of past emotional experiences. Learning/conditioning has been shown by Eric Kandell and other neuroscientists to occur as biochemical changes stored at the receptor and cellular level. Modulation of receptors at nodal points by the various neuropeptides regulate which memories, perceptions and sensations readily percolate across synapses up the neuroaxis to emerge as conscious thought and which get suppressed in the subconscious or unconscious mind. The subconscious mind is located, not only in the back of the brain, but through the network of peptidergic interconnections spanning the autonomic ganglia, end organs, immune system and even the skin. THE UNCONSCIOUS MIND IS YOUR BODY!!

That the psychosomatic network has shared common components--- the peptide ligands and their receptors--- which use the same language, sending and receiving information without necessarily having a hierarchical control or command priority has interesting implications. The mind has potential access to every molecule and cell of the body through the psychosomatic network. Behavior takes place at the level of the whole organism, the sum of all decisions, conscious and unconscious, which are constantly being made from moment to moment. Because of the network rather than hierarchical organization of our bodyminds, old unconscious traumas lodged deep in the body (the intestines, for example which are a very rich source of neuropeptides) can "take command" and lead us to irrational or destructive behaviors. The ideal state for perfect health is one of free-flowing communication, integration, wholeness.

Mindbody techniques such as meditation, yogic breathing, conscious movement and massage are powerful tools for enhancing consciousness and enlightening "dark", "blocked-off" areas of the psychosomatic network where pain and disease-causing trauma can persist in the form of "somatoemotional cysts" (as John Upledger has called them). Stanley Krippner has documented how virtually all healing rituals in the world have concommitants of strong emotional release. I believe it may now be possible to scientifically study how mind-body techniques can intervene in the psychosomatic network to exert their healing effects in order to optimize their effectiveness. For example, we now know that the floor of the fourth ventricle in hindbrain contains the "breathing center", a small group of neuronal cell bodies, dendritic and axonal processes that contain virtually every neuropeptide that has been carefully sought there. A large literature reviewed by my colleague Joanna Hill describes how various neuropeptides applied to this center alter the depth, frequency and other variables of breathing. Various forms of conscious breathing must surely alter the secretion of peptides from this center into the cerebrospinal fluid, which ultimately bathes the entire spinal cord through its central canal, effecting and transforming mood states and physical events throughout the bodymind. I am proposing more research on **how,** not whether, mind-body interventions improve health, being already convinced from my own personal experience that they do. An astonishingly large percentage of mainstream medical practice has not been scientifically proven, and I am not proposing--as some have--that complementary mind-body medicine be held to a higher standard of proof before it may be utilized by the many who can benefit.

Selected Bibliography

1. "Opiate Receptor: Demonstration in Nervous Tissue." Candace B. Pert and Solomon H. Snyder. *Science.* March 9, 1973 (vol. 179)
2. "Neuropeptides and Their Receptors: A Psychosomatic Network." Candace B. Pert, et al. *Journal of Immunology.* August, 1985 (vol. 135, no. 2).
3. "Neuropeptides Are Chemoattractants for Human Monocytes and Tumor Cells: A Basis for Mind-Body Communication." Michael Ruff and Candace B. Pert. In *Enkephalins and Endorphins: Stress and the Immune System,* edited by Nicholas P. Plotnikoff, et al. Plenum Publishing Corporation: New York, 1986
4. "The Wisdom of the Receptors." Candace B. Pert. *Advances,* Summer 1986 (vol. 3, no. 3). Also appeared in Noetic Sciences Review, Spring 1987. Institute of Noetic Sciences, Sausalito, CA
5. Small cell carcinoma of the lung: macrophage-specific antigens suggest hemopoietic stem cell origin. Michael Ruff and Candace Pert *Science* 225: 1034-1036 1984.
6. Octapeptides deduced from the neuropeptide receptor-like pattern of antigen T4 in brain potently inhibit human immunodeficiency virus receptor binding and T-cell infectivity. Candace Pert, et. al. *Proc. Natl. Acad. Sci. USA* 83: 9254-9258, 1986.

IMAGINING IS ACTING: EXPERIENCED PHYSICAL ACTION AS THE BASIS FOR IMAGINATION AND LINGUISTIC KNOWLEDGE

Kiyotaka Miyazaki,
Cognitive Psychology, Associate Professer, School of Human Sciences, Waseda University, Japan.

Cognition has its basis in the body, as the human being lives and experiences, as Varela, Thompson, & Rosch have strongly asserted in their book (1991). Although the relevance of bodily experience to cognition has been shown in some areas by some authors (e.g. Johnson, 1987 in some linguistic concepts), it still remains to be explored in many areas of cognition. This paper tries to shed light on how the body works with imagination. Imagination is selected as the topic here partly because imagery has been, and is widely believed to be, the phenomenon deep in the mind of the human being, detached from the body experience. I believe that the imagination even works, if not exclusively, on the bodily experience of the human being. It is asserted here that experienced physical action of the embodied human being plays a vital role in the generation of imagery. The more actively the embodied human being conducts the experienced physical action in the imagination process, the more fertile imagery that is generated, and in consequence, the more deeply the world is understood. Some evidence sup-

Experienced physical action	Behavior
Lived and experienced	Observed from the outside
With intention	Inferred intention
Reciprocal relation with meaning of the world	Induced by stimulus
Felt from the inside	Seen from the outside

Experienced physical action vs. Behavior

porting these assertions will be presented from the practical usage of imagery in theatrical activities and education.

EXPERIENCED PHYSICAL ACTION

First, the maining of the term 'experienced physical action' should be explicated briefly. It should be distinguished from the term behavior as commonly used in psychology. Behavior, as observable by the outside observer, is the set of movements of the body in the sense of natural science. Experienced physical action, on the other hand, is lived, experienced by the human being as agent, though it is possible for it to be shared, co-experienced by other persons intersubjectively. It has characteristics as follows.

It is intentional. Experienced physical action is always with the agent's purpose, goals, and intentions. These are only inferred from the outside after the behavior is accomplished. In experienced physical action, these are lived and experienced by the agent, explicitly sometimes, tacitly other times.

It is situated. Experienced physical action is always in a concrete spatio-temporal situation. With purpose, goals, and intentions, the agent acts on the world, or more precisely on the meanings of the world surrounding the agent. And it is acted upon by the world. Behavior, on the contrary, is only caused by stimuli, the physical characteristics of the world, not by the meaning of the world.

It is of the whole body. It is experienced with all the sensory modalities, both exteroceptive and interoceptive. Contrary to the behavior seen from the outside, it is first of all felt from the inside.

ACTION CREATES IMAGINATION: STANISLAVSKI'S METHOD OF PHYSICAL ACTION

Though many experimental studies have been conducted on imagery in these three decades, only a few of them treated the relationship between imagery generation and the agent's experienced body (e.g. Sayeki, 1987, on the mental rotation task and Finke,

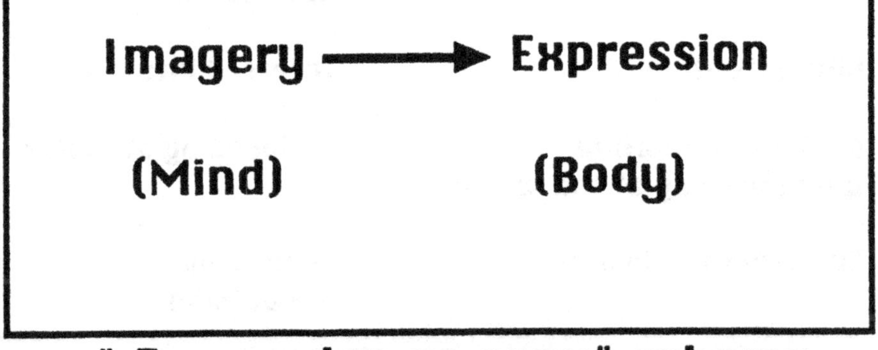

" Expression as copy" scheme

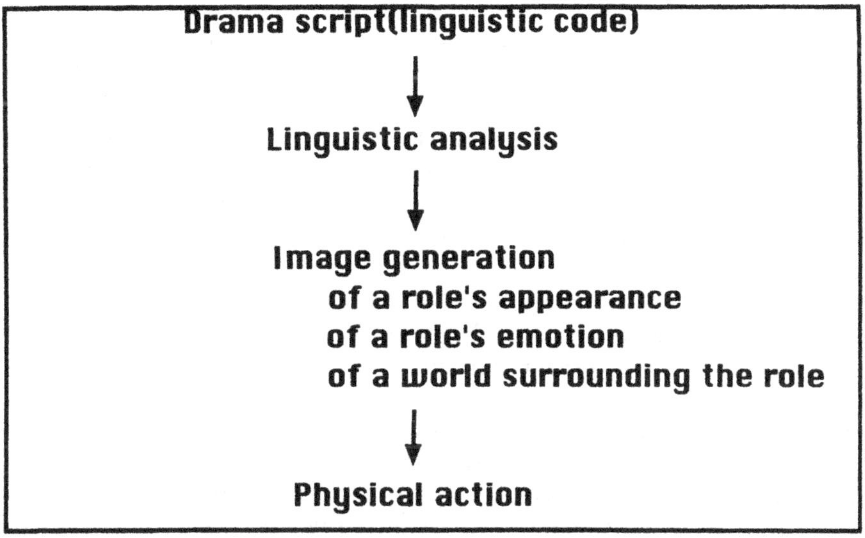

"Expression as copy" scheme in dramatic performance

1990, on creative imagery). We will concentrate on analyzing a special case of imagination, artistic expression. In particular, dramatic expression and its application to education will be discussed here.
In not only dramatic expression but artistic expression in general, it has been ordinarily assumed that expression is the result of imagery. First comes imagination generated deep in the inner mind, then it is acted out, resulting in expression of the outer body. This scheme can be described as "expression as copy theory", as expression is thought to be the copy of imagery. The good performer copies the inner image well, and the poor performer copies it badly. This scheme is a reflection of the mind-body dualism which has been permeating our culture deeply.

In dramatic expression, this scheme can be extended as follows. First comes a drama script given in a linguistic code. The actor analyzes the script linguistically and generates imagery of the assigned role's appearance, his emotion, and the role's world. Finally he externalizes this imagery with his body.

Konstantin S. Stanislavski (1863-1937), the great Russian actor/director, opposed this view (Stanislavski, 1979,1980). He devoted his life to finding a way how an actor can live a role on the stage, experiencing the emotion of the role and the imaginary world surrounding the role. He finally developed in the last days of his life the method which he called "the method of physical action". His method of physical action can be schematized as 'from action to imagery'. Instead of a fine analysis of a drama script, he gave an actor a rough sketch of the context in which the role was to be placed together with the purpose of the role. For example, a protagonist is standing at the door of the room in which is his lover whom he has not met for a long time. And then the actor is asked to explore how the role could be acted in the situation. Open the door? How? Deliberately or in a hurry? By acting out in various ways, the actor started elaborating the given situation: Imagining things surrounding the role and feeling emotion as the felt role. If you opened the door deliberately, how do you feel about your lover? How do you feel if you do it in a hurry? Is the door easy to open or not? How does the role feel? Hurrying to meet her? Trying to disguise his feelings? Acting is exploring by the actor his imagination of the world and his emotion as he lives his role.

The nucleus of his thought is best shown in one of the basic practices he proposed for the actor to enrich his imagination: The method of non-object action. In this practice, the actor is asked to perform a simple action like drinking a cup of water without a cup. He has to act on the object, which does not exist, as he would on a real one. He should perform the components of action, i.e., gripping the cup, lifting the cup, touching the rim of the cup with his lips, and drinking water, all with coherence.

It should be emphasized that this performance is distinguished from mime. The actor should not imitate real action. The actor does not need to communicate what he is doing to the audience. The actor is required to concentrate his attention on an object which does not exist as if it really does exist. He is asked not only to move his fingers, hands, and arms to touch and move it, but also to move his head and his eyes to see it as he would with a real object. The actor is asked to see and feel it as he sees and feels a real object.

If physical action here is not an imitative one, what is it? The answer is that it is an exploratory action. In ordinary action with an object acted upon, the action is performed automatically. You do not need to look at your action in detail. Without an object, however, it becomes necessary for the actor to attend to his action, to scrutinize carefully how to act, how to move his body piece by piece. As physical action is intentional and situated, looking for how to act is exploring what the object acted upon is like for him. By exploring how to act, the actor explores information about the characteristics of the objects which enables him to act. As the object is not a real one, information has to be generated from the actor's memory. In another words, imagery of the object is generated. In this case, memory is not of articulated knowledge of the object but of tacit knowledge which only the actor's body knows.

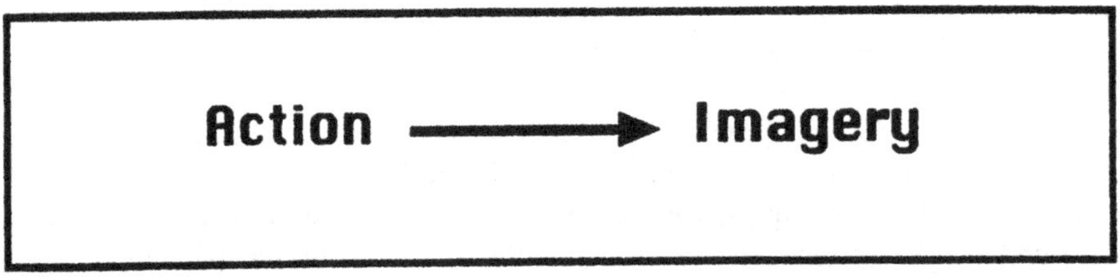

Stanislavski's method of physical action :The first approximation

Take a case of drinking a cup of water as an example. First, the actor tries to grip a cup. This action is an exploration of the information about the type of grip of the cup. In adjusting the motion of fingers and hand, the actor looks for the shape and the tactile feeling of the surface of the grip. As his body knows how it has touched and felt the various types of grip in earlier encounters with cups, action facilitates the generation of information on the grip. He somehow generates information about the grip. Information thus generated orients his next exploratory action. Using this information as a basis, he now grasps a cup and tries to lift it. In doing so, he explores how heavy it is as he holds it in his grip. Information generated here provides the basis for the next action, touching the rim of the cup with his lips, and so on.

There is a reciprocal circle between exploratory action and information generated in this process. Exploratory action facilitates the actor in generating information, and the generated information guides and orients the next exploratory action. In the method of non-object action, the scheme is rather simple. Generated information is about the object acted upon. However, this reciprocal process underlies the whole process of dramatic expression in the case of Stanislavski's method of physical action. Here, the scheme becomes a little bit complicated, though basically the same. The action becomes a complicated one, not like drinking a cup of water, but like revenging his dead father. However, it is still exploratory in nature, and comprised of many simple actions. Generated information is no longer on the single object, but on the world surrounding one's role, or on what the world is like for the role. Emotions and ainner thoughts about the role are also generated from the reciprocal circle. The first schematization for Stanislavski's method should be revised with respect to the reciprocal circle between exploratory action and the generated information scheme. Viewed from inside, this circle is the process of imagery generation. Viewed from outside, this circle is the process of expression. Here, imagery and expression are not separable. These are the two aspects of the same process. The process can be termed as the expression=imagery process.

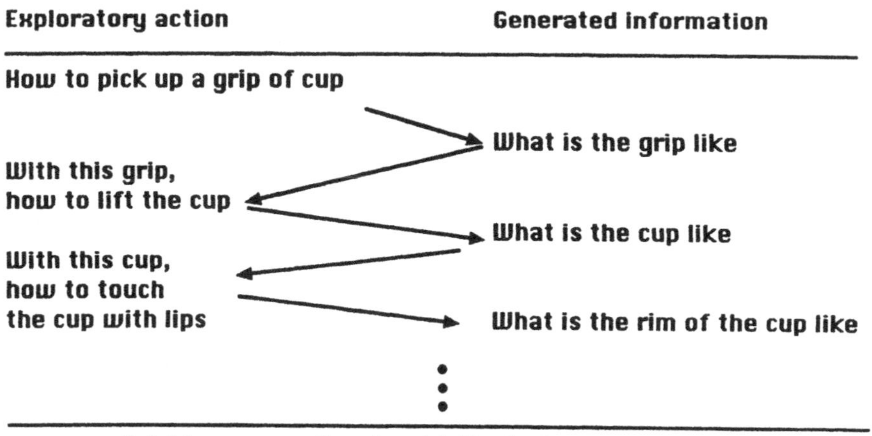

Drinking a cup of water: Method of non-object action

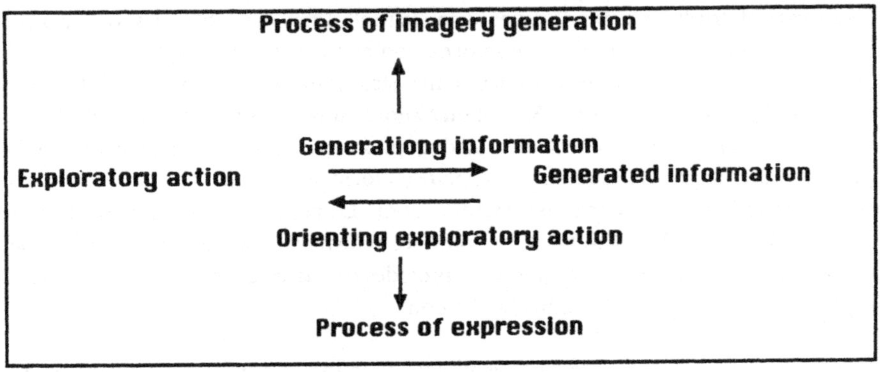

"Expression = imagery" scheme

Understanding the world by being-thrown-into it

The expression=imagery process makes it possible for the agent to enrich his understanding of the world. This can be shown well in its application to education. Here, one such application which is named as "learning by being-thrown-into" will be analyzed. In Japan, Toshiharu Takeuchi, a director, has developed Stanislavski's thought further (Takeuchi, 1975). He has argued that the way people relate to the other people, the world and themselves has its root in the way people experience their bodies. He has developed many techniques to change these relations on the horizon of bodily experience. Toshiko Toriyama, a primary school teacher, adapted his thinking to childrens' learning in primary schools and developed the method of "learning by being-thrown-into".

This is a sort of dramatic method of teaching, but contrary to its western counterparts (e.g. Bolton, 1984), the emphasis is not on the script. Nor is it just a role taking practice. Children are asked to throw themselves into objects of the learning, such as animals, flowers, and even the inanimate objects like rocks and trashes. They generate the imagery of the objects and the world surrounding them and live as the objects do by acting as these objects and feel with their bodies as if they were these objects.

What is the aim of this learning? It is for children to live as these objects, to know how they exist in the world from inside themselves, and to deepen their understanding of them. Someone might ask if there are "insides" for objects like animals and flowers. He might ask if it makes sense to talk about knowing them from the inside. Certainly not, for the inanimate objects like rocks. These doubts are another reflection on mind-body dualism, though. Everything, even the inanimate, exists in the world in relationship with other things. What children do here is to re-experience the relationship objects have with other things in their experienced action, in their action in and towards the world. Someone might still ask if it makes any sense to talk about learning as, even if everything exists in relationship with others, it is impossible for us human beings to really re-experience the relationship. What children can do is simply to imagine it as they can not have any correct answers to learn. The apparent answer to this question is: Yes, children can not learn one true relationship. However, they can explore many possibilities on the way relationships exist by their exploratory action in being-thrown-into activities. In action, it is possible for them to shed new light on the way objects exist beyond the knowledge that they have already acquired.

What do children do to throw themselves into objects in order to learn? As in the case of Stanislavski's method of non-object action, they are committed to experienced physical action. And this action is exploratory too. They do not imitate the movements and the appearances of objects.

To throw themselves into the objects, they first generate the intention that the objects have. Then, they start exploring in their action the way that the objects relate to the surrounding world. In their exploration, they generate information on the aspects of the world which must be relevant to the objects.

Here, contrary to the case of the method of non-object action, children do not have the experience of the interaction with the world that the objects experience as their own. However, they must have had similar experiences. They try to conduct such interactive action upon the world. Some might fit, some might not. They are looking for the one which has a verisimilitude for them. Towards these aspects of the world, they keep acting, and elaborating their image of the world. Through this reciprocal circle, they understand how the objects relate to the world, and how the objects exist in the world. Though it might not be a true one as mentioned before, it would be a discovery of a new aspect for them, one beyond their previous understanding.

Take a throwing-into-a flower of orchid, for example. First, children felt an intention which an orchid flower might have growing and blossoming. With this intention in mind, they explored, in action, how an orchid flower related to the world. In this case, two aspects of the relationship seemed important to children. One was the relationship with the ground, or the gravity of the earth. Children's up and down motion with their knees, bending and straightening, shows that they explored how the orchid grows against the pull of gravity of the earth. The other was the relationship with the surrounding space. Their rotating motion with their arms extending shows that they explored how the orchid expands into the surrounding space in its growth. With such exploratory actions, they generated the imagery of the orchid's world with both gravity and surrounding space, and got an understandiong of how the orchid grows.

The children's poetry which they wrote after this learning activity gives us some hints about what they learned in it. One child wrote as follows.

How is the orchid flower growing, extending to the sky from a seed?

Is it growing without awareness of its growing, as I felt? Or, is it growing with awareness?

From a bud, it is formed into a curious shape, more and more a curious shape, and flower leaves resulted.

Where did such a mysterious phenomenon come from?

What do the colors of the flower leaves mean?

Who made them?

Veining and patterns on the flower leaves, their shapes.

Who made them?
I felt somehow vaguely the way one flower grew up into the sky with various motions.

This child generated many questions that she did not have before. It shows how children deepen their understanding of the orchid through this expression=imagery activity.

The expression=imagery scheme: Is it generalizable?

In this paper, the expression=imagery scheme was presented to show that imagery should not be treated as a phenomenon detached from experience of the body. Exploratory physical action plays a vital role in the imagery process. However, as the topics analyzed here are restricted to the specific area of theatrical expression, it remains unsolved whether or not this scheme is applicable to the other forms of the expression, and to mental imagery in general. There is a possibility, I believe, that this is the case.
Take a drawing as an example. In ordinary thinking, drawing is a copy of mental imagery. It might not be correct. There is an exploratory action in drawing a picture. In this case, the exploratory action is performed on canvas as the painting action of hands, arms and a brush as their extension. Painters explore how they see the object, generating information on the object that is relevant to them in the painting action on the canvas. Through such an exploratory action, a drawing is produced on the one hand, and imagery is generated on the other hand.
How about mental imagery in general? Take a look at a simple case like recalling what you saw yesterday. Even in such a simple task, there is a component of exploratory action, though tacit. You have to explore where you were and what you saw yesterday. Though it is not an actual action, but a possible one, it is still an exploratory action. More generally, as Neisser (1976) argued in his Gibsonian account of perception, exploratory action and its planning are the essential components of perception. It must be so, I believe, with mental imagery in general, i.e. with perception of possible worlds.

References

Bolton, G. (1984). *Drama as Education: An Argument for Placing Drama at the Centre of the Curriculum*. Essex: Longman.
Finke, R. (1990). *Creative Imagery: Discoveries and Inventions in Visualization.* NJ:Lawrence Earlbaum Associates.
Johnson, M. (1987). *The Body in the Mind: The Bodily Basis of Meaning, Imagination, and Reason.* IL: The Chicago University Press.
Neisser, U. (1976). *Cognition and Reality.* CA:Freeman.
Sayeki, Y. (1987). Anthropomorphic Epistemology. Paper presented at the third International Imagery Conference.
Stanislavski, K. (1979). *Building a Character.* London: Methuen (First published in 1950).
Stanislavski, K. (1980). *An Actor Prepares.* London: Methuen (First published in 1937).
Stanislavski, K. (1979). *Building a Character.* London: Methuen (First published in 1950).
Stanislavski, K. (1980). *Anerparts* (e.g. Bolton, 1984).

Takeuchi, T. (1975). *Kotoba ga Hirakareru Toki (When Voices are Opened)*. Tokyo:Shiso-no-Kagaku-Sha.

Varela, F., Thompson, E., & Rosch, E. (1991). *The Embodied Mind: Cognitive Science and Human Experience*. MA: MIT Press

THE BODY AS LIVED: RECOGNIZING LIVED BODY DISRUPTION IN ILLNESS

S. Kay Toombs, Ph.D.,
Associate Professor, Philosophy Department, Baylor University, Waco, Texas USA

Abstract: The phenomenological account of lived body (the body I "exist" rather than "have") discloses the body as orientational and intentional locus in the world, thus giving valuable insights into the dynamic relation between body, mind, world, self, others. Emotional and physical disorders engender a profound disruption in the lived body, a disruption that includes a transformation of the surrounding world, important changes in the perception of time, an altered relation with body, disturbances in social interaction, and threat to self integrity. An understanding of lived body disruption can have important application in the clinical context in devising effective therapies.

My interest in the phenomenology of the body has grown out of my own experience as a person living with neurological disease. In 1973, at the age of 30, I was diagnosed with multiple sclerosis. Since that time I have lived with progressively disabling illness and have become increasingly aware that the prevailing biomedical model of disease not only captures little of the actual experience of illness but also gives an incomplete account of bodily disorder. In conceiving the body to be a materialistic, machine-like entity, the biomedical model not only separates mind from body but also radically de-emphasizes the dynamic relation that exists between body/mind/world/self and others -- a relation that must be taken into account when understanding and responding to the needs of patients [1].

In what follows, I shall argue that the notion of embodiment provides profound insights into the illness experience, as well as suggesting therapeutic approaches that transcend narrowly conceived disease categories.

I would like to begin by briefly explicating the notion of embodiment. As an embodied being, I do not simply "have" a body, as I "have" a house, a car or a pet. Rather, I "live" or "exist" my body [2] [3]. In the English language it is difficult to express this relation of bodily existing in a non-dualistic fashion. If we use the words "live" or "exist" in reference to the body, we would be likely to say, "I exist in my body," or I live in my body" -- language that suggests some kind of a separation between an encompassing physical entity and a subject within. In reality, however, there is no such separation. Rather than being an object of the world, my body as I live it represents my particular point of view on the world. In this respect the lived body is not the objective, physiological body that can be seen by others (or examined by means of various medical technologies) but, rather, the body that is the vehicle for seeing.

Under normal circumstances one does not perceive one's body as a separate entity. Indeed, the body is largely taken-for-granted and ignored. When I read a book, for instance, my attention is directed to the meaning of the text. I am not explicitly aware of the functioning of my eyes or my brain in focusing on and interpreting the print. Nor do I pay attention to the position of my limbs as I sit in the chair, or the coordinated movements of my arm and hand that accomplish the turning of the page. In all my activities the lived body is given only implicitly as the center of reference for my world, a center which is indicated but never grasped as such [2].

As the center of reference for my world, the lived body orients me to the world around by means of my senses and positions the world in accord with my bodily placement. The world and the objects within it are experienced as invitations to my body's possible actions according to my particular aims and projects [3].The pen on the table is perceived as "an instrument for writing" or, perhaps, as "an object to be replaced in the drawer." Depending on my intentions, the desk inside my office represents "a location for working," or alternatively "an obstacle to wheel around in order to get to the door." The surrounding world is always grasped in terms of a concrete situation. Contained in the action of reaching for the cup is the intention to bring it to one's lips. One reaches for the cup in order to drink from it.

Points in space do not represent merely objective positions but rather they mark the varying range of one's aims and gestures. For example, a narrow passageway represents a "restrictive potentiality" for my body, requiring a modification of my actions [3] [4]. I must perhaps turn sideways in order to make my way through it. The passageway may also limit my actions not only because of its physical dimensions but because it appears threatening, ominous, impossibly claustrophobic [6].

As the locus of one's intentions, the lived body represents the realm of existential possibilities. A leg is more than a limb -- it is the possibility of strolling along a path with one's friend, of running up a flight of stairs to reach a desired destination. The body is also the ground of one's future possibilities continually influencing and delimiting life choices.

The lived body is also an expression of personal identity. Each of us has a unique body style -- ways of moving, gesturing, laughing, speaking -- that is peculiarly our own. When I check my appearance in a mirror, or catch sight of my reflection as I move past a store window, I immediately recognize not only a physical body, or even my physical body, but rather I see an embodied being who is ME and nobody else. Moreover, I live my body in ways that express my particular being-in-the-world. If I am an aggressive person, I live my aggression in my posture, in the tensing of my muscles, in the tone of my voice, in the rapidity of my heartbeat.

Lived Body and the Experience of Illness

Illness transforms the experience of embodiment engendering a profound disruption in the lived body -- a disruption that includes a profound sense of bodily alienation, a change in the physiognomy of the surrounding world, the loss of corporeal identity and the loss of self integrity [1] [5] [7].

The experience of bodily alienation begins with a radical change in the everyday taken-for-granted relation with one's body. Rather than being unreflectively lived, the body intrudes itself into consciousness becoming the unwilling object of one's attention. This shift in consciousness occurs whenever one becomes aware of alien sensations such as pain, fatigue, or dizziness, or an unexpected alteration in function. One must stop whatever one is doing in order explicitly to focus on the body. If one has trouble grasping a cup, for instance, one is preoccupied with the ineffectiveness of one's hand or the clumsiness of one's fingers. Pain or extreme fatigue anchor one's awareness in the body preventing involvement in other-directed activities.

The loss of bodily taken-for-grantedness is accompanied by a profound sense of vulnerability. In illness one recognizes in a concrete way that the body is a neurophysiological organism with its own nature and, more importantly, that there is a symbiotic relation between body and self. Whatever happens in and to MY BODY also necessarily happens to ME. When speaking of ourselves when we are sick we do not say "My body has cancer, my body is going to die."

If I realized nothing else when I received the diagnosis of multiple sclerosis, I recognized that the disorder in my body threatened every aspect of my existence. The experience of illness is always the experience of "having" and "being had." I not only "have" an illness, it also has me in its clutches [8].

This sense of vulnerability is not a pathological fear. Rather it arises in the sensed experience of embodiment and the overt recognition that my body "has its own nature, functions, structures, and biological conditions, since it embodies me ... I am exposed to whatever can influence, threaten, inhibit, or benefit my biological organism" [9].

Illness is also experienced as the concrete loss of possibility. In the context of everyday life, symptoms are not experienced as abstract signs indicative of a particular disease. Rather, they are the inability to engage the world in ways that are important and meaningful. A severe headache is more than an uncomfortable sensation. It is the "inability to" concentrate on the book I am reading, the impossibility of carrying out a personal project. Depression is not only a certain kind of affective disorder, it is the impossibility of energizing oneself to perform the most mundane of tasks. The loss of existential possibility may take the form of future threat. What will I do if my headaches continue? Will I be able to work at my job? How can I stand it if this sense of hopelessness never ends? [10].

Illness discloses the intimate relation between body and the surrounding world. Not only is it the case that one's capacity to interact with the world changes according to one's physical and mental state, but the dimensions of the surrounding world change according to the the range of possible movements [11] . When one is unable to leave the house or one's room, what was formerly regarded as near (work, the neighbor's house, the doctor's office) is now impossibly far. A problem with the body is a problem with the environment. From a wheelchair the ticket counter at the airport is unreasonably high -- all the transactions with the person behind the counter take place at the level of one's ear. Regardless of its measurement in inches, a curb is as high as a wall if one is in a wheelchair or cannot lift one's foot to clear it.

The physiognomy of the world may also change in the sense that the world feels different. We not only act in the world, we dwell in the world. We know this well in everyday life when the world is transformed for us in times of grief or in moments of great joy. If I am depressed, the world appears grayer than hitherto; when I grieve the colors of the leaves on the trees are muted, the laughter of others unseemingly loud. Depending on one's situation the world may appear unusually effortful, impossibly stressful. Allow me give a concrete example that illustrates a transformation in space: Recently I was crossing the wide open plaza outside the university library when my battery operated wheelchair stopped dead in its tracks. I was surrounded by a sea of concrete embedded with decorative pebbles, marooned in the middle of a flat, completely open area with no trees, no lampposts, no benches within reach. There was no-one in sight. The nearest "object" was the building but I couldn't crawl the distance because of the hard, uneven surface of pebbled cement. And I was incapable of getting to the telephone in my van because it was parked several hundred yards away down a short flight of steps. The space of the plaza which a minute before had been open, spacious, sunny, bright, now appeared deserted, bare, ominous. And in an instant I was referred back to my malfunctioning body, the magnitude of my physical limitations and my dependence upon mechanical devices to negotiate space.

In curtailing the ability to pursue plans and projects and in affecting personal relationships, illness necessarily disrupts the various roles that we occupy -- father, breadwinner, professional, wife. This significant disruption in role is experienced as a profound threat to self-integrity. In our culture there is great emphasis on the importance of "doing" rather than "being." A person's worth is judged according to his or her capacity to produce (to be useful) or the ability to achieve a certain professional status. The inability to carry out one's role inevitably causes one to feel diminished in person, as well as in body.

Changes in body style may also be profoundly alienating. Each of us has a unique way of walking, talking, gesturing with which we are comfortable and which we recognize as peculiarly our own. To lose this accustomed manner of bodily being is to lose one's sense of bodily identity. This loss is particularly profound when the alteration of body style is permanent.

In my own experience of neurological disease, I have found it difficult to identify with changed and changing patterns of movement. When I see myself on a home video, I experience a sense of puzzlement. I catch myself wondering not so much whether the body projected on the screen is my body but, rather, if the person in the video is really ME. At the same time, if I see pictures of myself when I was walking, or leaning on a cane, I find it hard to remember how it was to be that person or, even, who I was when I moved like that.

Since the body represents one's self expression to others, societal judgements with respect to body style directly affect one's sense of personal worth [12]. I live in a culture that places great emphasis on physical fitness, sexuality, productivity and youth -- an ideal that is associated with a particular bodily physique. Consequently, there is little tolerance for physical difference or deviation from the ideal. When strangers observe that I am in a wheelchair, they make immediate judgements about me as a person. In noting my physical incapacities, most conclude that I am dependent on others and unable to engage in professional activities. In perceiving my mobility is limited, others conclude that my intellect must be likewise affected. In my presence, strangers frequently address questions to my companion and refer to me in the third person. "Where would SHE like to sit? Does SHE want us to move this chair?" (This invariably happens when we go through airports. When we wheel up to the security barrier, the airport employee looks directly at me and then turns to my husband and says "Can SHE walk at all?" We now have a standard response. My husband says "No, but SHE CAN talk!")

The loss of upright posture is particularly significant [13]. Just as an infant's sense of autonomy and independence grows with the ability to stand up and venture into the world unaided, so there is a corresponding loss of autonomy with the loss of upright posture. There is more than metaphorical significance to such expressions as "looking down on" and "looking up to." In "looking up to" others, and being "looked down on," one experiences oneself as inferior. This response is not pathological but is grounded in embodied experience. For example, when seated in a wheelchair one is approximately three and a half feet tall. From this perspective a person who is standing is experienced as unusually tall in relation to oneself. One must bend one's head back and look up to speak to them. This bodily experience of being situated below people who are much taller than oneself inevitably causes one to feel like a child again surrounded by very large adults.

Emotions such as fear and shame also exemplify the global disruption of the lived body. Shame is an integral element of disordered embodiment - a non-rational response to a change in bodily being.

At one level (to use Sartre's terminology) shame is the experience of "The Look." One sees oneself through the eyes of the Other in a negative fashion [2]. It is important to emphasize here the felt dimension of the interaction with others. We directly experience the Other's responses (facial expressions, gestures, averted eyes), it is not simply a matter of what I think you feel about me.

Shame is also present in the frustration of intentionality. The inability to interact with the world is not only an experience of loss "I can no longer do" but diminishment "I must depend on others to do for me" and further "I should be able to do for myself."

In neurological disorder shame also manifests itself as an increase in the severity of physical symptoms. In the experience of "the Look" an already existing tremor invariably intensifies, spastic limbs become more rigid, difficulty controlling movement becomes more pronounced.

For instance, on the occasion of receiving my doctoral degree, I was to be seated on the stage. I was still able to walk a few yards with assistance and the day before the ceremony went to the auditorium with a colleague to practice negotiating the steps onto the stage. In the empty auditorium I managed quite well. But the next day -- in the concrete Look of an audience of 20,000 eyes, my leg refused to move. It was not just that I was embarrassed at my awkward gait, rather, my leg was paralyzed.

As Van den Berg and others have noted, shame is not a purely psychical quality, it is "that which encompasses the body, encases it like a garment." Shame always has a physical meaning [6]..

Emotions such as fear and anxiety incorporate profound changes in embodiment. After suffering a serious accident in my wheelchair, I was diagnosed with post traumatic stress disorder. This disorder was not simply "in my head" as opposed to "in my body." I experienced it concretely as a suffocating shortness of breath, a rapidly escalating heart rate, a tautness in my shoulders, back, and neck, and a terrifying recurring physical sensation of flipping over backwards.

I also lived my disorder as a frightening, and very real, transformation in the physiognomy of the world. Flat surfaces menaced since they concealed hidden obstacles, modest curb cuts were too steep to negotiate, uneven surfaces inherently dangerous. The world threatened in a myriad of ways.

Moreover, I no longer trusted my tacit "knowing how" to negotiate space. Just as the person on two feet unreflectively judges how high to lift a foot in order to clear a curb, so the person who lives in a wheelchair unthinkingly performs the physical movements necessary to negotiate space. The wheelchair is incorporated into the body in such a way that one intuitively allows for the width of the chair when going through a doorway, in the same way that a tall person intuitively allows for her height in bending her head. My accident compromised this embodied knowledge. My senses could no longer be trusted. Rather than being an extension of body, my wheelchair appeared as an object that could cause me great harm. Since my chair is the means by which I live and interact with the world, this experience of alienation profoundly affected my ability to carry out all my daily activities. My recovery depended upon directly addressing all these disturbances that transformed not only my bodily being but my being-in-the-world.

In sum, then, the notion of embodiment provides the important insight that illness is experienced as a global disorder that represents a profound disruption of the lived body. In terms of the traditional biomedical model, the dynamic relation between body/mind/word/self/others is de-emphasized. The illness experience is thus truncated, or split into different categories (physical, mental, psycho/social) that, to the patient are distressingly artificial.

Although construing multiple sclerosis as a purely physical disorder of the central nervous system and explicating the changes in terms of demyelination may give valuable information about the effect of the disease process on my brain and spinal chord, such an account captures nothing of my particular experience of M.S. Nor can my experience be relegated to the purely psycho/social aspects of disease. Lived body disruption is not simply a psycho/social aspect of my illness, in a fundamental way it IS my illness. The notion of embodiment provides a holistic account of illness that is vital in the therapeutic endeavor:

For instance, addressing the profound experience of bodily alienation involves instituting therapies that enable patients to co-exist with their malfunctioning bodies in ways that are integrative. I have in mind the kind of work that is being done by Jon Kabat-Zinn and his colleagues that teaches patients to move their attention back in to the body (rather than trying to escape from it), to re-establish a sense of connectedness in spite of ongoing disorder, thus providing a renewed sense of unity and control.

Paying explicit attention to the altered relation between body/world means intervening to change the experience of space. In this respect, knowing how the world feels to a particular patient --threatening, empty, desolate, or perhaps restrictive, effortful, demanding, is important information that can direct therapy.

Attending to embodied emotions expands the therapeutic focus to include the myriad of ways in which emotions are lived.

Preserving or re-establishing self integrity becomes central to the goal of healing in debilitating illness, recognizing that the sense of self worth is intimately related to bodily identity, existential possibility, worldly involvement, and the relationship with others.

And lastly healing may be conceived as the process of recovering body and mind (not necessarily through cure of disease) but in the sense of re-instituting wholeness through restoring lived body unity.

References

Toombs SK. (1992) *The Meaning of Illness: A Phenomenological Account of the Different Perspectives of Physician and Patient.* Dordrecht, The Netherlands: Kluwer Academic Publishers.

Sartre J-P. (1956) *Being and Nothingness: A Phenomenological Essay on Ontology.* New York: Pocket Books.

Merleau-Ponty M. (1962) *Phenomenology of Perception.* London: Routledge and Kegan Paul.

Schutz A. and Luckmann T. (1973) *The Structures of the Lifeworld.* R. M. Zaner and H. T. Englehardt, Jr. (trans.) Evanston Illinois: Northwestern University Press.

Toombs SK. (1994) "Disability and the Self" in TM Brinthaupt and RP Lipka (eds.), *Changing the Self: Philosophies, Techniques and Experiences.* New York: SUNY Press.

Van den Berg JH. (1955) *The Phenomenological Approach to Psychiatry.* Springfield, Illinois: Charles C. Thomas.

Toombs SK. (1995) Healing and Incurable Illness. *Humane Medicine* 11: 98-103.

Toombs SK. (1995) "Sufficient Unto the Day: A Life with Multiple Sclerosis" in SK Toombs, D Barnard, RA Carson (eds.) *Chronic Illness: From Experience to Policy.* Indiana: Indiana University Press.

Zaner, RM. (1981) The *Context of Self: A Phenomenological Inquiry Using Medicine as a Clue.* Ohio: Ohio University Press.

Toombs, SK. (1990) "The Temporality of Illness: Four Levels of Experience." *Theoretical Medicine* 11: 227-241.

Toombs SK. (1995) "The Lived Experience of Disability." Human Studies 1995; 18: 9-23.

Goffman E. (1963) *Stigma: Notes on the Management of Spoiled Identity.* New Jersey: Prentice Hall.

Straus E. (1966) *Phenomenological Psychology, Selected Papers.* E. Eng (trans.) New York: Basic Books.

Kabat-Zinn, J. (1990) *Full Catastrophe Living.* New York: Dell Publishing.

Made in the USA
Monee, IL
05 November 2026

67385384R00098